JOHN ADAMS

John Adams: A Research and Information Guide offers the first comprehensive guide to the musical works and literature of one of the leading American composers of our time.

The research guide catalogs and summarizes materials relating to Adams's work, providing detailed annotated bibliographic entries for both primary and secondary sources. Covering writings by and interviews with Adams, books, journal articles and book chapters, newspaper articles and reviews, dissertations, video recordings, and other sources, the guide also contains a chronology of Adams's life, a discography, and a list of compositions. Robust indexes enable researchers to easily locate sources by author, composition, or subject.

This volume is a major reference tool for all those interested in Adams and his music, and a valuable resource for students and researchers of minimalism, contemporary American music, and twentieth-century music more broadly.

Alexander Sanchez-Behar is Associate Professor of Music Theory at Texas A&M University, Kingsville, USA.

ROUTLEDGE MUSIC BIBLIOGRAPHIES

RECENT TITLES

COMPOSERS

John Adams (2020)
Alexander Sanchez-Behar

Isaac Albéniz, 2nd Edition (2015)
Walter A. Clark

William Alwyn (2013)
John C. Dressler

Samuel Barber, 2nd Edition (2012)
Wayne C. Wentzel

Béla Bartók, 3rd Edition (2011)
Elliott Antokoletz and Paolo
Susanni

Alban Berg, 3rd Edition (2018)
Bryan R. Simms

Leonard Bernstein, 2nd Edition
(2015)
Paul R. Laird and Hsun Lin

Johannes Brahms, 2nd Edition (2011)
Heather Platt

William Byrd, 3rd Edition (2012)
Richard Turbet

John Cage (2017)
Sara Haefeli

Frédéric Chopin, 2nd Edition (2015)
William Smialek and Maja
Trochimczyk

Miles Davis (2017)
Clarence Henry

John Dowland (2019)
K. Dawn Grapes

Edward Elgar, 2nd Edition (2013)
Christopher Kent

Gabriel Fauré, 2nd Edition (2011)
Edward R. Phillips

Alberto Ginastera (2011)
Deborah Schwartz-Kates

Fanny Hensel (2019)
Laura K.T. Stokes

Gustav Holst (2011)
Mary Christison Huismann

Charles Ives, 2nd Edition (2010)
Gayle Sherwood Magee

Quincy Jones (2014)
Clarence Bernard Henry

*Alma Mahler and Her
Contemporaries* (2017)
Susan M. Filler

Bohuslav Martinů (2014)
Robert Simon

*Felix Mendelssohn Bartholdy,
2nd Edition* (2011)
John Michael Cooper with
Angela R. Mace

Olivier Messiaen, 2nd Edition (2017)
Vincent P. Benitez

Claudio Monteverdi (2018)
Susan Lewis and Maria Virginia
Acuña

*Nikolay Andreevich Rimsky-
Korsakov, 2nd Edition* (2015)
Gerald R. Seaman

Gioachino Rossini, 2nd Edition (2010)
Denise P. Gallo

Pëtr Il'ich Tchaikovsky (2019)
Gerald R. Seaman

Ralph Vaughan Williams (2016)
Ryan Ross

Giuseppe Verdi, 2nd Edition (2012)
Gregory W. Harwood

Richard Wagner, 2nd Edition (2010)
Michael Saffle

Anton Webern (2017)
Darin Hoskisson

GENRES

*Blues, Funk, R&B, Soul, Hip Hop,
and Rap* (2010)
Eddie S. Meadows

Chamber Music, 3rd Edition (2010)
John H. Baron

Choral Music, 3rd Edition (2019)
James Michael Floyd

*Church and Worship Music in the
United States, 2nd Edition* (2017)
Avery T. Sharp and James
Michael Floyd

Ethnomusicology, 2nd Edition
(2013)
Jennifer C. Post

*Film Music in the Sound Era,
Volumes 1 & 2* (2020)
Jonathan Rhodes Lee

Free Jazz (2018)
Jeffrey Schwartz

The Madrigal (2012)
Susan Lewis Hammond

The Musical, 2nd Edition (2011)
William A. Everett

North American Fiddle Music
(2011)
Drew Beisswenger

*Popular Music Theory and
Analysis* (2017)
Thomas Robinson

The Recorder, 3rd Edition (2012)
Richard Griscom and David
Lasocki

String Quartets, 2nd Edition (2011)
Mara E. Parker

Women in Music, 2nd Edition (2011)
Karin Pendle and Melinda Boyd

JOHN ADAMS
A Research and Information Guide

ALEXANDER SANCHEZ-BEHAR

THE ROUTLEDGE MUSIC BIOGRAPHIES

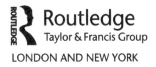

Routledge
Taylor & Francis Group

LONDON AND NEW YORK

First published 2020 by Routledge

2 Park Square, Milton Park, Abingdon, Oxon OX14 4RN

605 Third Avenue, New York, NY 10017

Routledge is an imprint of the Taylor & Francis Group, an informa business

First issued in paperback 2022

Library of Congress Cataloging-in-Publication Data
Names: Sanchez-Behar, Alexander, author.
Title: John Adams : a research and information guide / Alexander Sanchez-Behar.
Description: New York : Routledge, 2020. | Series: Routledge music bibliographies | Includes bibliographical references and index.
Identifiers: LCCN 2019055770 (print) | LCCN 2019055771 (ebook) | ISBN 9781138055803 (hardback) | ISBN 9781315165714 (ebook)
Subjects: LCSH: Adams, John, 1947—Bibliography.
Classification: LCC ML134.A345 S26 2020 (print) | LCC ML134.A345 (ebook) | DDC 016.78092—dc23
LC record available at https://lccn.loc.gov/2019055770
LC ebook record available at https://lccn.loc.gov/2019055771

ISBN: 978-1-138-05580-3 (hbk)
ISBN: 978-1-03-233643-5 (pbk)
DOI: 10.4324/9781315165714

Typeset in Minion
by Apex CoVantage, LLC

Contents

Acknowledgments

This book would not have been possible without the support of many individuals. I wish to express my gratitude to:

My wife and children, Neda, Sofia, and Cyrus, who showed utmost patience throughout this project. To my late father, Fernando Sánchez Barroso, my mother, Dorothy Behar, and my siblings, Laura and Daniel, for their unwavering love and encouragement. To Music Editor Genevieve Aoki and the entire Routledge team for their belief and support of this book. To my former colleague at Ashland University, Dr. Christina Fuhrmann, for her mentorship during the initial stages of my academic career. To my dissertation advisor at Florida State University, Dr. Michael Buchler, for making music theory more inviting and teaching me to think outside the box. To fellow Adams scholars Drs. Rebecca Jemian and Timothy A. Johnson, for supporting my research aims by reading article drafts and providing feedback during professional conferences. To my colleagues at Texas A&M University-Kingsville, including Drs. Darin Hoskisson, Joseph E. Jones, and Greg Sanders, for reading the first draft of this proposal. To the James C. Jernigan Library at Texas A&M University-Kingsville, chiefly Agueda Gonzales from the Interlibrary Loan Department and Library Director Bruce Schueneman, for assisting in finding any and all materials related to the production of this book. And to Dr. Steven J. Corbett, Director of the Texas A&M University-Kingsville Writing Center, for awarding me a grant to assist me in the completion of this book.

Preface

It is often said that musical studies woefully lag behind composers' lives and their creative output. Only a handful of living composers receive immediate recognition from the public and scholarly community that helps generate numerous publications about their life, musical style, and compositions. The American contemporary composer John Adams, born in 1947, warrants such attention.

Research and information guides such as this strive to offer more than a utilitarian means of compiling relevant sources with basic annotations. My guide aims to consolidate and contextualize a diverse body of writings that explore John Adams and his musical works. Critical commentary on recent writings and musical trends relevant to the study of John Adams are deemed essential. When called for, my discourse will describe available literature using concise reports typical for a research guide. Conversely, when a specific study merits greater attention for its importance or relevant content, I provide a lengthier annotation in the style of a critical review. Though more considerable in length, these responses, helping to situate the first-of-its-kind research guide on Adams, identify fertile and uncharted areas worthy of further exploration. Additionally, these annotations help the reader navigate much of the recent literature, highlighting the significance of various topics and findings, noting discrepancies in analytical segments and other matters, and reframing studies in relation to current musicological and theoretical research and other modes of investigation at the present time. Lastly, the annotations collate vital information for each musical work within a single library source.

While I strive to incorporate as many sources from as diverse a corpus of literature as possible, it would seem unrealistic to give the impression of an exhaustive compendium. In many respects, scholarly studies of Adams's music are at a budding stage, and as such, new books and articles appear in print on a yearly basis. Regarding concert and recording reviews, I aim to integrate a representative sampling from various music critics while omitting most reviews that duplicate much the same sentiment without adding additional content. The *Klinghoffer* controversy is a notable exception, where it is important for readers to weigh the opinions of various critics and scholars in order to be informed and arrive at their own conclusion. The discography of Adams's recordings expands and updates Thomas May's discography from his 2006 book *The John Adams Reader*. Some of the earlier recordings available in LP or cassette format are not readily accessible to listeners while newer recordings of the same works are widely available for purchase.

Given the modest number of sources on Adams compared to early twentieth-century composers from the Routledge series, I find it more practical to arrange chapters by types of sources in publication, rather than adopting Adams's compositions into individual chapters in chronological order. Moreover, many of the available publications could not be easily categorized in this alternative manner because they entail studies of several different musical works.

The sources in this guide were located using a variety of databases of bibliographic information, including WorldCat, Répertoire International de Littérature Musicale (RILM), ProQuest, JSTOR, Grove Music Encyclopedia, online resources for Adams's official webpage, Boosey & Hawkes, online discography databases, and numerous others. The majority of scholarly studies appear in English, though there are select publications in other languages, most notably German—additional information on foreign language sources appears along with their bibliography entries. I suspect that Adams's collaboration with the Berlin Philharmonic as composer-in-residence, as well as his recent recordings with this world-renowned orchestra will continue to spark new interest in Germany and throughout Europe, and in time bolster Adams scholarship further.

Introduction

It seems only a handful of contemporary composers today garner the level of recognition known to John Adams. Reports from The League of American Orchestras indicate that Adams's symphonic works are the most frequently programmed in American concert halls among living American composers. The New York Philharmonic, the San Francisco Symphony, the Los Angeles Philharmonic, and other prestigious national and international orchestras feature one or several of Adams's works during their concert seasons. His operatic works have earned Adams even more attention. Opera houses from around the world invest all of their resources to create new productions of his operas. It is easy to understand why there is much enthusiasm: his musical works are sure winners, guaranteeing a home run for professional ensembles marketing upcoming concert series. His operatic works are polarizing and elicit a visceral response from critics and audience members. Upon witnessing the world premiere of Adams's first opera, *Nixon in China*, *New York Times* critic Donal Henahan summarized his scathing review, declaring, "Mr. Adams does for the arpeggio what McDonald's did for the hamburger, grinding out one simple idea unto eternity." *The Death of Klinghoffer*, considered the most contentious opera in modern times, bears parallels not unlike the riot that sparked following Stravinsky's premiere of his 1913 ballet *Le Sacre du printemps*. Adams's premiere was plagued by protests and bomb threats. For over two decades now, the sensitive nature of his second opera has incited a slew of people, ranging from religious groups such as the Jewish Information League, to politicians like Rudy Giuliani, to the renowned musicologist Richard Taruskin, to protest the opera on claims of anti-Semitism. Clearly, his music evokes, or rather *demands*, a strong reaction or commitment from those who care to listen.

Stemming from this growing fascination for Adams's music are numerous studies that attempt to probe deeper into the score in search for answers. The earliest publications that introduce readers to Adams and his music appear in the form of newspaper articles. Reviews of Adams's premieres and subsequent performances abound in the *New York Times*, the *Los Angeles Times*, and the *San Francisco Chronicle*, in particular. It is no coincidence that Taruskin published his review against Adams's *Klinghoffer* in the *New York Times* considering that this newspaper boasts the largest circulation in the United States. Similarly, the *Los Angeles Times* plays a significant role in promoting Adams's music since the composer has collaborated for years with the Los Angeles Philharmonic and its former music and artistic director Esa-Pekka Salonen and his successor, Gustavo Dudamel. Ever since Adams relocated to Berkeley in the early 1970s, the *San Francisco Chronicle* has been a proponent of their resident composer, who has shared a longstanding professional relationship with the San Francisco Symphony and its music director, Michael Tilson Thomas.

Another early printed source consists of concert program notes and compact-disc liner notes. Some of the program notes are written by critics such as Michael Steinberg, performers like Sarah Cahill, fellow composers such as Ingram Marshall, and others by Adams himself. Searching for program notes from decades ago is challenging and at times yields little reward due to their superficial descriptions of newly composed works. Immeasurably more useful are the liner notes written by Adams, many of which appear, in part or full, in his official website: www.earbox.com. These firsthand synopses shed light on Adams's titles and offer information deemed germane to Adams's compositional process. Clearly, vivid titles such as *Grand Pianola Music* and *A Short Ride in a Fast Machine* remain an enigma to listeners without anecdotal information. A select number of compact-disc liner notes are released with open access online through the music database Discogs as well as Chandos Records.

Scholarly publications on the subject of Adams's musical aesthetic and compositions begin to appear in print during the late 1980s. Brent Heisinger's study on American minimalism attempts to define the musical style in common to minimalists and categorize their influences and aesthetic aims. Dan Warburton's study addresses minimalism as a whole by familiarizing readers with common compositional techniques along with new music terminology applicable to minimalist composers and their works. During this decade Adams's *Nixon in China* (1987) receives much interest, and its bold subject, combined with dramatic twists and turns enlaced in a minimalist style, afforded the composer international acclaim.

Resulting from his successes from *Harmonium*, *Harmonielehre*, and *Nixon in China*, a growing number of publications appear on the study of Adams's works in the 1990s. In 1990 the late K. Robert Schwarz's "Process vs. Intuition in the Recent Works of Steve Reich and John Adams" brings to light an important dichotomy in the development of the minimalist aesthetic. Namely, Adams's works from the 1980s onward exemplify a freer and more dramatic approach to writing within the minimalist vein, inspiring John Rockwell's coinage of Adams's style as postminimalist.

Theoretical studies emerge during the 1990s in the form of dissertations, theses, and scholarly articles. In 1991, Timothy A. Johnson publishes the first dissertation devoted solely to Adams's works. Johnson's music-theoretical study dispels the notion that minimalist music defies analysis by providing tools for understanding Adams's harmony in works beginning with *Phrygian Gates* and culminating with *Nixon in China*. In 1993,

Rebecca Burkhardt publishes her dissertation on Adams's musical development from 1978 to 1989. Burkhardt illustrates through score study how Adams's style shifted away from early minimalist traits to incorporate chromaticism, polyharmony, and a faster harmonic rhythm. In 1998, Paul Reed Barsom publishes a dissertation on large-scale tonal structure in Adams's works between the years 1977 and 1987. Lastly, in 1999, Catherine Ann Pellegrino publishes her study of formalist analysis in the context of Adams's minimalist style, noting its inherent postmodern tendencies.

Musicological studies from the 1990s focus predominantly on *Nixon in China* and *The Death of Klinghoffer*. David Schwarz's 1992–93 journal articles examine *Nixon* using concepts from Freudian and Lacanian psychoanalytic criticism to highlight parallels between psychic and musical structures. In 1993, Stephan Martin Prock investigates the underlying subtext of musical and dramatic discourse in *Nixon*. In 1995, Matthew Daines writes about parody, gender politics, and cultural representation. In a different study, Daines explores layers of meaning in the final act of the opera while describing how Adams forgoes traditional operatic conventions. In her 1998 dissertation, Linell Gray Moss explores the role of the opera chorus as a character in Adams's second opera. In 1998, Brandon Joel Derfler publishes his thesis whose central premise is motivated by the assertion that Adams's compositions diverge from process-driven minimalist works and can be more aptly approached using Arnold Schoenberg's notions of organicism.

Throughout Adams's career, we also find numerous interviews initiated by radio hosts, music critics, scholars, and public relations staff or other members from professional ensembles. This medium is of great importance to the study of Adams's works since it opens a window into the composer's perspective of his works and other relevant aspects of his career. Furthermore, the nature of his interviews far exceeds anecdotal conversation. His interviews present Adams as a candid and introspective composer, often sharing one or more germinating ideas on the creation of his new works, inadvertently prodding scholars for further investigation of his notions of symmetry, the role of intuition, postminimalism, and many other subjects that served as the central topic for published studies.

Scholars in the twenty-first century have benefited from earlier publications, and the result is a growing body of publications. The most ambitious studies include Timothy A. Johnson's 2011 book on *Nixon in China* and Thomas May's 2006 compilation of writings on the composer. Johnson's book blends analytical aspects of Adams's opera with historical and political perspectives. Johnson employs newer analytical tools, such as neo-Riemannian theory, to describe Adams's signature harmonic progressions written in a minimalist idiom. Thomas May's collection of writings touches upon portraits of the artist, his musical works, Adams's collaborators and interpreters, and critical reception of his works. A lengthy section on the critical reception of Adams's music contains numerous writings on the *Klinghoffer* debate.

The literature on Adams from these last two decades displays a wider range of topics and analytical approaches. Analytical and musicological studies of individual works are being published with greater frequency. Some of these studies focus on Adams's works that helped define his earlier musical style, while other recent articles and dissertations are forging new territory with in-depth studies of Adams's musical works from the 1990s onwards—including studies of the Chamber Symphony, *Lollapalooza*, and *Naive and Sentimental Music.* Scholars are beginning to consider social, cultural, and gender aspects of Adams's works, paying special attention to his operas. Aspects of otherness and orientalism have been considered. A number of scholarly studies on cultural memory, practices, and collectivity appear in print, as do interdisciplinary studies of Adams's works and an investigation of religious principles, like salvation, as a central theme in his music. The direction of studies in musical analysis is deepening while also adapting to Adams's stylistic development over the course of his career. We now find studies of Adams's works on subjects such as rhythm and meter, musical form, counterpoint, musical processes, symmetry, and harmonic transformations. Other emergent approaches touch upon musical aesthetics, semiotics, narrative studies, appropriation of minimalist techniques in film music, and the new field of ludomusicology.

Scholars today will also benefit from Adams's 2008 autobiography, *Hallelujah Junction: Composing an American Life.* Though his memoir is intended for a wide readership ranging from the general public to music enthusiasts and connoisseurs alike, scholars will value having the most complete biographical content available in print and other germane information on his musical works and their reception, his thoughts on other composers all the way from Bach to Milton Babbitt and Frank Zappa, and commentary on a host of topics relevant to his own musical style, jazz influences, and asserting the composer's voice within the scope of minimalist music to form a unique style. It would not be an understatement to claim that many of the scholarly writings on Adams would not been come to fruition without background information directly from the composer. Timothy A. Johnson's writings on harmony are motivated, in part, from an interview with Adams himself. My own writings are also informed by Adams's explanations of his compositional process and musical influences.

Among the types of literature published on Adams in the relatively short span of his ongoing career, there are studies geared specifically for performers as well as conductors. The kind of readership intended in work-specific studies will overlap between scholars and practicing musicians. Furthermore, there are studies that address performance issues in Adams's piano works, concertos, and various other works. Select general solo repertoire studies that furnish performance commentary and annotated bibliographies also cite Adams's relevant works, as do studies on orchestral programming, wind band and orchestra, modern percussion ensemble, clarinet repertoire, baritone and bass arias from Adams's operas, and trumpet excerpts. Some of the practical studies tie in a study of Adams's stylistic development. In one such study, Thomas May asserts that Adams's development can be charted in string music.

A future stage of research on Adams will undoubtedly include sketch studies. At present time, Adams houses his working sketches and completed manuscripts in his own personal archive. Obtaining facsimiles of Adams's scores and sketches is not feasible in most instances, though musicologist Alice Miller Cotter has had the good fortune to view and study Adams's library and subsequently publish her dissertation on compositional practice and revision of his operas. Future scholars engaged in this mode of research will be faced with what sketch studies means and what its boundaries are in an age of computers. His personal library should also bring to surface a few unpublished compositions for further study, such as his 1970 Piano Quintet.

   One of Adams's principal artistic aims throughout his career, that of creating music that invites the listener without subjecting them to a cerebral rite of passage, reflects a late postmodern aesthetic that imbues his minimalist techniques with a Romantic aesthetic. During his formative years as a composer, Adams came to the realization while listening to Wagner's opening bars of "Dawn and Siegfried's Rhine Journey" that Wagner cared deeply about the expressivity of his art. What Adams found in the Romantics was a way out of the dreary attitude expressed in Milton Babbitt's 1958 article "Who Cares if You Listen?" that pervaded concert music and music conservatories during Adams's early years. Recent publications demonstrate how far the study of music and instruction of composition has moved from Babbitt's mode of thinking. The steady increase of studies on the music of Adams and other minimalists reveals that scholars have embraced Adams's post-postmodern style. Adams, now in his 70s, does not appear to be slowing down his output as a composer and conductor. Similarly, scholarly research about his life and music will continue to thrive. This is just the beginning.

Historians like to see what happened to European classical music in the wake of Wagnerism as a reaction against its suffocating hegemony. They'll say that the animal energy of Stravinsky and the compressed, hyper-expressive lyricism of the Viennese School—Schoenberg, Berg, and Webern—were responses to or reactions against the vast influence that Wagner's music, indeed his whole ideology, exerted on the field of musical and dramatic aesthetics.
   But it's been my experience that creative artists don't make art in the negative mode. One doesn't suffer through the agonies of forging a personal language, of wresting something out of nothing simply to react against an oppressive father figure or merely to rebel against a received way of doing things. Granted, rebellion in a young artist can be a tonic, a productive and liberating energy. But works like *Le Sacre du printemps*, *Pierrot Lunaire*, and Ives's Forth Symphony emerged not because the composers were reacting against Wagner and his epigones but rather because the composers *needed* to make them, because the times had changed and a new expression, a new way of experiencing the world, was called for.
                              (from Adams's autobiography *Hallelujah Junction:*
                                   Composing an American Life, 102–3)

1

Chronology of John Adams's Life

1947   Born in Worcester, Massachusetts, on February 15, 1947 to Carl John Vincent Adams and Elinore Mary Coolidge. Both parents were amateur musicians. Carl, who was a clarinetist, provided John's earliest musical training.

1950   Family moved to Woodstock, Vermont.

1954   Moved to Concord, New Hampshire, prompted by a new job for Carl at an industrial hardware company.

1955   Began clarinet lessons with his father.

1956   First lessons in composition, harmony, and theory under the instruction of an unnamed teacher from Saint Paul's Preparatory School.

1960   Clarinet lessons under the tutelage of Felix Viscuglia, bass clarinetist of the Boston Symphony.

1962   Joined the New Hampshire State Hospital Auxiliary Orchestra. John Adams composed and conducted an unpublished suite for string orchestra. Attended a summer music camp in western Maine where he conducted Schumann's Piano Concerto.

1964–65   Private studies in conducting lessons from music director Mario di Bonaventura, who was a student of Nadia Boulanger and Igor Markevitch. Studied keyboard harmony and analysis from Luise Vosgerchian, student of Nadia Boulanger and professor at Harvard University. Met Walter Piston, professor emeritus of Harvard University. During his senior year in high school, Adams was a member of the Greater Boston Youth Symphony.

1965–69   Undergraduate studies at Harvard University. Instruction in harmony from
           Harvard professor Elliot Forbes, followed by studies in counterpoint from David
           Del Tredici. In 1966 Adams joined the Boston Symphony Orchestra as a substitute
           and performed the American premiere of Schoenberg's *Moses und Aron*. In
           the summer of 1966 Adams heard Duke Ellington perform in person. In 1967
           Adams, together with actor John Lithgow, staged six performances of Mozart's
           Le Nozze di Figaro. As a junior, Adams was the student conductor of Harvard's
           Bach Society Orchestra, which performed repertoire ranging from Bach to
           contemporary music. Adams wrote a letter to Leonard Bernstein about the state
           of contemporary music and the cognitive dissonance it was eliciting for Adams.
           Bernstein responded shortly thereafter of his own struggles with avant-garde
           music. In 1968 Adams declined an invitation to attend the conducting program
           at Tanglewood. During his last years at Harvard, Adams took private lessons in
           composition and analysis from Earl Kim and Leon Kirchner, both of whom were
           Arnold Schoenberg's pupils. In spring 1969 Adams performed Piston's Clarinet
           Concerto at Carnegie Hall in a concert performed by the Harvard-Radcliffe
           Orchestra. Adams completed his undergraduate studies in July 1969.

1969   Began graduate studies in composition at Harvard University.

1970   Married Hawley Currens, music teacher in Boston schools and daughter of a
           cardiologist.

1971   Completed a master's degree in composition at Harvard University. Shortly
           after graduation, Adams and his wife moved to Berkeley, California. During
           this time, Adams worked as an apartment building manager assistant and
           subsequently at a warehouse in Oakland called Regal Apparel.

1972   Adams's friend Ivan Tcherepnin informed Adams of a music-composition
           vacancy at the San Francisco Conservatory. Adams joined their faculty and
           remained there for ten years. In addition to his teaching duties, Adams was
           responsible for directing the New Music Ensemble for the school's series of
           New Music concerts.

1974   Adams and Hawley Currens divorced. Adams relocated to San Francisco.

1978   Became New Music Advisor for the San Francisco Symphony.

1981   Met his future wife, Deborah O'Grady, at the New Music America Festival.

1982   Resigned from his teaching post at the San Francisco Conservatory. In the
           same year, Adams received a three-year commission as composer-in-residence
           with the San Francisco Symphony Orchestra through the Meet the Composer
           Orchestra Residencies Program.

1983   Met Peter Sellars at the Monadnock Music Festival.

1984   Adams's daughter, Emily Davis Adams, was born on May 30, 1984. The week
           after Emily's birth their family moved back to Berkeley.

1985   In December Adams was introduced to Alice Goodman by Peter Sellars, to begin working on *Nixon in China*

         Adams's son, Samuel Carl Adams, was born on December 30, 1985.

1988   Won the Grammy Award for the Best Classical Contemporary Composition for *Nixon in China*.

         Named Creative Chair of the Saint Paul Chamber Orchestra. He served with this orchestra for two years as conductor and advisor.

         In the spring Adams accepted an invitation to be resident of the American Academy in Rome. While living in Rome, Adams received an invitation to attend the Third International Music Festival for Humanism, Peace and Friendship Among Nations to be held the same year in Leningrad, Russia. While at the festival Adams formed a friendship with composer John Cage. At the Festival, the Lithuanian orchestra performed *Harmonielehre*.

1992   Began integrating musical ideas from Nicolas Slonimsky's 1947 compendium titled *Thesaurus of Scales and Melodic Patterns* in his compositions. Adams acknowledged this influence on his works since the Chamber Symphony. The two composers formed a friendship at an unknown date after Slonimsky had moved to California.

1993   Won the Royal Philharmonic Award for his Chamber Symphony.

1995   Won the Grawemeyer Award for Violin Concerto.

1997   Won the Grammy Award for the Best Classical Contemporary Composition for *El Dorado*.

2002   Received a commission to write a work in memorial of September 11. He titled the work *On the Transmigration of Souls*.

2003   Won the Pulitzer Prize in Music for *On the Transmigration of Souls*.

         Received a commission to write for the opening of the Walt Disney Concert Hall in Los Angeles. Adams titled his new composition *The Dharma at Big Sur*.

         Appointed Artist in Association with the BBC Symphony Orchestra and composer-in-residence at Carnegie Hall.

2004   Won the Grammy Award for the Best Classical Contemporary Composition for *The Transmigration of Souls*.

         Won the Nemmers Prize in Composition from Northwestern University. Along with the cash award and a performance of the composer's works with the Chicago Symphony Orchestra, Adams was granted a residency with the Northwestern University Bienen School of Music.

2007   Awarded the Harvard Arts Medal, a distinction for demonstrated achievement in the arts by a Harvard alumnus.

2008   Recipient of the Honorary Doctor of Music degree from Northwestern University.

2009   Won the National Endowment for the Arts Opera Honors Award.

Appointed Inaugural Creative Chair of the Los Angeles Philharmonic.

Recipient of the Honorary Doctor of Music degree from Duquesne University.

2012   Recipient of the Honorary Doctor of Music degree from Harvard University.

2013   Recipient of the Honorary Doctor of Music degree from Yale University.

2015   Recipient of the Honorary Doctor of Music degree from the Royal Academy of Music.

2016   Named composer-in-residence at the Berlin Philharmoniker.

2017   Awarded the San Francisco Opera Medal.

2019   Awarded the Erasmus Prize by The Netherlands' Praemium Erasmianum Foundation for exceptional contribution in the arts.

2

Writings by Adams

1.   Adams, John. *Hallelujah Junction: Composing an American Life*. New York: Farrar, Straus and Giroux, 2008.

Adams's autobiography is an important source for scholars of minimalist music and musicians wishing to explore the composer's life and works. The layout and content are intended to be autobiographical in nature, and to that aim, the book represents the most comprehensive source available. Adams's memoir details his family history, recounting his earliest musical experiences as a child in his family's Winnipesaukee Gardens, where they had a dance hall that was frequented by touring musicians and other important figures such as Duke Ellington. Adams's personal anecdotes reveal his love of jazz and classical music from an early age. He gives accounts of learning to play the clarinet under the tutelage of his father. He contemplates a transformative moment at an early age when his third-grade teacher read a biography of Mozart to his class. That moment planted the seed that would blossom into a life of musical composition.

During his college years as a music major at Harvard University, he experienced a dialectical opposition between his love of popular music and the academic avant-garde that pervaded universities across the country. Adams recalls corresponding with Leonard Bernstein about his frustrations over the state of contemporary classical music. This conflict of musical forces proved pivotal in the formation of Adams's compositional style, rooted in the continuum of classical or art music, though with a popular, minimalist aesthetic that appealed to the composer. Adams pinpoints the composers who were most influential to his own development, among them the American modernist Charles Ives and one of the pioneers of musical minimalism, Steve Reich.

Adams's autobiography details how, upon graduating from college, he made the decision to relocate to the West Coast. He elaborates on all of the menial jobs he worked at until he was serendipitously sought out by the San Francisco Conservatory to teach music composition classes. Working as a composer and directing the New Music Ensemble at the conservatory helped Adams nurture his career and lead to an important commission with the San Francisco Symphony.

In the remainder of his autobiography, Adams discusses the personal history and motivation for writing each composition from beginning stages to completion. He provides an insight into the creative process and the development of his compositional style. Overall, Adams gives readers a glimpse into his career and his thoughts on music in a way that no other writer could.

2.   ____. *John Adams Official Website.* Accessed December 21, 2018. www.earbox. com.

Adams's official website offers extensive notes on his musical works in greater detail than his publisher, Boosey & Hawkes. In addition to program notes, one can hear sample audio clips of his works, view portions of opera productions on video (from *Nixon in China* and *Doctor Atomic*), find featured recordings for sale, and for select works, hear video interviews with the composer. Adams's website has undergone notable changes in layout and content over the years. For about a year circa 2010, Adams wrote a series of posts on a wide range of musical subjects in a blog format, and readers added comments and expressed their views. The posts had a light and humorous nature, and their subjects were often about Adams's neighbor as well as the French novelist Marcel Proust. These posts no longer appear in Adams's website. At present, the composer features news items on his Twitter and Facebook accounts. Recent updates to the website have resulted in less content along with an updated list of Adams's works, though readers can access previous versions of his official website through the online internet archive *Wayback Machine* (https://archive.org/web).

3.   ____. "Three Weeks to Go for Doctor Atomic." *NewMusicBox* (September 9, 2005). http:// www.newmusicbox.org/articles/Three-Weeks-to-Go-for-Doctor-Atomic.

Adams writes a reflection piece on his impressions of *Doctor Atomic* rehearsals in anticipation of the world premiere. This article is not duplicated in Adams's official website. Adams explains the process of revising the score after hearing baritone Gerald Finley sing musical selections. Adams composed the opera using detailed MIDI mockups of the instrumental parts before finalizing the work. The composer touches on many issues related to vocal composition and shows an aversion toward the operatic tradition that uses loud orchestration and makes text largely unintelligible. Instead, Adams opts for some amplification of the voices with the aid of sound designer Mark Grey. He brings to attention a major scene that was left out of the final opera, consisting of a phone conversation between General Groves and an army doctor. Adams believes the dramatic and musical form was complete without this scene (Alice Miller Cotter provides additional information on this scene in her 2016 dissertation). Additionally, Adams discusses text setting and being loyal to a librettist's artistic aims while reflecting on his previous collaborations with Alice Goodman and June Jordan. Last, Adams reveals plans for a *Doctor Atomic* symphony, not with the structure of a suite or musical extracts, but rather recomposing the opera into a symphony in the same vein as Hindemith's *Mathis der Mahler* symphony.

3

Books

4. Botha, Marc. *A Theory of Minimalism*. London: Bloomsbury Academic, 2017.

Botha contends that a valid definition of minimalism cannot be reduced to a set of traits or musical works no matter how inclusive the given parameters. Instead, minimalism is thought of as a way of comporting towards two kinds of minimum: infinitesimal, or least possible, and parsimonious, or least necessary. Botha adopts the work of phenomenologist Roman Ingarden to form the argument that minimalism "intensifies and clarifies access to the real" (xiv). With his precedent in mind, Botha explores seven distinct concepts: historical intermittency, the encounter, objecthood, the real, radical quantity, lessness, and minimum. Rather than ascribing the genesis of minimalism from an enclosed chronological perspective, Botha presents a transhistorical theory of minimalist aesthetics.

Botha's study presents a wide overview of the minimalist aesthetic, examining numerous composers and musical works. Steve Reich's works receive noticeably more attention than Adams's, though Botha's brief discussions of the latter offer novel ideas. In the fifth chapter, "Quantity: On the Radicality of Minimalism," the author explores continuity as sustained sound or silence, and calculation as seriality or incremental repetition. He employs Kant's notion of sublime in regards to works such as Adams's *On the Transmigration of Souls*, for its emergence of "dynamics of thought and the imagination, which allow us indirectly to confront and overcome the fear-arousing objects and situations" (133). Botha asserts that Adams's listing of missing persons in *On the Transmigration of Souls* acts as "markers for place, identity, and the crossing of personal, interpersonal and cultural histories" (134).

In the sixth chapter, Botha devotes a section to Adams's *Shaker Loops* entitled "The Minimalism of Waiting." He explores the religious underpinnings of the work's title. The music bears an aesthetic akin to Quaker spirituality and through the exclusion of excess. The author concurs with K. Robert Schwarz that Adams's work shifted emphasis from audible process to an intuitive grasp of musical form. He details the principal characteristics of each of the movements. Botha creates a narrative of *Shaker Loops* that manifests a search for clarity: "Shaking and Trembling" provides anticipatory energy, "Hymning Slews" provides calm fluidity, "Loops and Verses" gives rise to energetic outbursts characterized by dramatic shifts and sudden halts, and "Final Shaking" returns to "the shimmering recapitulation" (146).

5.　Everett, Yayoi Uno. *Reconfiguring Myth and Narrative in Contemporary Opera: Osvaldo Golijov, Kaija Saariaho, John Adams, and Tan Dun*. Indianapolis: Indiana University Press, 2015.

Everett's book explores four contemporary operas—by Golijov, Saariaho, Adams, and Dun—from the perspective that while the music and libretto constitute the initial source material, they operate in counterpoint to the director's production components, including choreography, lighting, props, and filmic projections. The author incorporates critical discourse from gender, cultural, literary, psychoanalytic, and media theories. In the realm of musical semiotics, Everett draws on the work of Robert Hatten and others to delve into how the music shapes one's own reading of operatic narrative in relation to other fields. Everett purports that contemporary operas diverge from earlier twentieth-century operas in that postwar operas employ non-linear forms of narrative—a point that Elise K. Kirk also makes in her 2001 book *American Opera*. Everett expresses that one of the central goals of her study is to understand how contemporary opera reconfigures familiar myths and narratives. According to Everett, Adams's subject evokes mythical or historical figures from other eras, namely, Robert Oppenheimer evokes the figure of Faust. As a preliminary to her investigation of *Doctor Atomic*, Everett traces the making of the opera.

The author's analysis of the opera is formed by a comparison of Peter Sellars's productions from the 2007 Netherlands Opera performance and the 2008 Metropolitan Opera with Penny Woolcock. Everett posits that as the opera unfolds, Adams's music becomes increasingly static while Sellars's libretto emphasizes timelessness over realism. The combined effect is associated with how viewers perceive mythological stories. Everett elaborates on how Adams's postminimalist style of writing aids in the process of shifting from the narrative to the mythical dimension of the narrative. In her examination of the arias, Everett provides an analysis of Oppenheimer's recitation of John Donne's Holy Sonnet XIV, entitled "Batter My Heart." Everett's analytical overview of Adams's arias (modeled after Edward Gollin's theoretical tool on double interval cycles) displays some of the most detailed analyses of Adams's opera music that appear in scholarly literature.

6.   Hutchinson, Mark. *Coherence in New Music: Experience, Aesthetics, Analysis.* London: Routledge, 2016.

The focus of Hutchinson's book is on finding coherence as a way of understanding musical works ranging from 1985 to 1995. The author centers on works from a number of prominent contemporary composers, including Adams, Kurtág, Ligeti, and Takemitsu, among others. Hutchinson examines Adams's Violin Concerto (primarily the first movement) throughout Chapter 3, entitled "Interaction, Analysis, Energy." Hutchinson provides an analysis of the textural layers that interplay throughout the movement and give the music a sense of continuity and energy. Several other key features are explored: tonality in contemporary works, Adams's unique approach to rhythm and meter enabled by the interaction of musical layers (foreground solo violin, accompanimental harmonies in the string, and countermelodies in the woodwinds). Hutchinson suggests a way of hearing textural strands and ties in his approach to semiotics—specifically, A. J. Greimas's concept of the semiotic square—allowing the music to dictate shifts and multiplicity to highlight focal points in musical textures.

7.   Johnson, Timothy A. *John Adams's* Nixon in China: *Musical Analysis, Historical and Political Perspectives.* Farnham, Surrey: Ashgate Publishing, 2011.

Johnson examines *Nixon in China* from an analytical perspective while taking into account historical and political circumstances during Nixon's visit to China in 1972. Johnson's book is organized in three main sections, the first of which examines how Adams and Goodman set the different scenes and landscapes with opposing views between American and Chinese characters. Johnson also examines the two official state ceremonial functions known as the official welcoming ceremony and the state dinner. The author discusses several other scenes, including Chairman Mao's study and the grand tour of China. The second part of Johnson's study explores the principal political figures: Richard Nixon, Pat Nixon, Henry Kissinger, Mao-Tse-tung, Chiang Ch'ing, and Chou En-lai. The third section of this book investigates nationalism and idealism between the United States and China, contrasting notions like American democracy versus the Chinese history of dynasties, Wall Street versus the Great Wall, and the manner in which these differences unfold throughout the opera.

Johnson implements various forms of musical analysis to elucidate important aspects of the opera and its characters. First, the author incorporates writings on metrical consonance and dissonance by Harald Krebs. Johnson asserts that beneath the surface structure of Adams's minimalist textures lie metrical irregularities in the form of continually shifting organizational schemes. The author contents that Adams frequently employs metrical dissonance to accompany the text. Another theoretical apparatus Johnson employs throughout the book is neo-Riemannian theory. He regards neo-Riemannian theory as complementary to his own common-tone index (stemming from his dissertation) since they both highlight the preservation of common tones. He uses the classical neo-Riemannian transformations for triads called *parallel, relative,* and *leading-tone exchange,* as well David Lewin's *slide* and avoids transformations for seventh chords on the basis that triads are the foundation of Adams's harmonic vocabulary. According to Johnson, Richard Cohn's influential work on hexatonic systems of neo-Riemannian progressions provides a useful way to connect Adams's harmonies that highlight mediant relationships. The author's application of neo-Riemannian concepts serves to identify characteristic chordal progressions between the characters in the opera. The harmonies accompanying Nixon, for instance, revolve around Cohn's Southern hexatonic system, which is at odds with the opening measures. On the other hand, the harmony from Premier Chou En-lai's final soliloquy revolves around major and minor triads drawn from the Northern hexatonic system.

8.   Kirk, Elise K. *American Opera.* Urbana and Chicago: University of Illinois Press, 2001.

Kirk explores the history of American opera, providing a survey that traces its origins from the second quarter of the eighteenth century toward the twenty-first century. The author provides a section in her chapter "Heroes for Our Time" on John Adams's expressive approaches to composing opera. Whereas Philip Glass draws from historical personages to compose his operas, Adams tends to favor contemporary plots and characters, focusing on the rise (and sometimes fall) of American heroes. According to the author, Adams molds minimalism beyond current trends by embedding coexisting musical styles, such as American popular music, jazz, and swing. Adams uses a saxophone quartet to evoke a romantic reverie between Pat and Richard Nixon. Kirk discusses aspects of the real-life characters and subject matter that appealed to Adams in making the opera—larger-than-life yet highly flawed personalities, along with the East meets West drama. The reception of this opera, as Kirk and others have noted, was enormous, usurping the throne held by Glass's *Einstein on the Beach.* Kirk provides some insightful citations from the collaborators of *Nixon in China* drawn from newspaper articles published shortly following the premiere in 1987. For instance, Alice Goodman debunks the notion that characters were portrayed with satirical gestures in one of these citations from the *New York Times.* These fresh and vivid impressions from the collaborators prove to be important to the understanding of the opera. Kirk also delves into Adams's second opera, *The Death of Klinghoffer,* which is composed in a newer and more contrapuntal style—as I note in my 2008 dissertation, this opera begins a new compositional path toward greater emphasis on foreground contrapuntal structures. Kirk explores the collaborators' approach to this opera as having emulated the formula of an oratorio, rather than composing an opera with a linear narrative. The chorus format plays a crucial role in this regard, as it exists outside of the timeframe of the opera. Kirk also elucidates some ideas regarding the musical techniques employed by Adams. She coins his newer style using the term "neo-sensualism," meaning greater chromaticism while maintaining minimalist figurations that act as accompaniment patterns.

9.   Machart, Renaud. *John Adams*. Arles: Actes-Sud, 2004. Translated by Thomas May in *The John Adams Reader: Essential Writings on an American Composer*, 386–95. Pompton Plains: Amadeus, 2006.

Thomas May translates a portion of Renaud Machart's book *John Adams* originally written in French. Machart begins by describing the overall feeling much of Adams's music seems to convey: as conductor Simon Rattle asserts in 1999, one of sadness and depth, with occasional works that serve as palate cleansers. The music archetype behind Adams's works, one that also reflects this elegiac sensibility, is Charles Ives's *The Unanswered Question*. Another connection to Ives's work can be traced back to Aaron Copland's *Quiet City*, which also features trumpet and English horn solos. The two works are related through their affinity to Walt Whitman's poem "The Mystic Trumpeter" in their qualitative nature. Machart shows readers that the way these two American composers, and later Adams, write for the trumpet complements Whitman's text from his poem. He purports the trumpet parts in *Tromba Lontana* and *Short Ride in a Fast Machine* portray the atmosphere expressed Whitman's verses. The role of the trumpet is central to other works by Adams, including the second movement of *Harmonielehre*, *The Wound-Dresser*, *On the Transmigration of Souls*, and *My Father Knew Charles Ives*. Machart believes these works portray the quality of floating elegies. The author discusses the floating quality of *Eros Piano* while asserting its harmonic language as a direct influence from Toru Takemitsu's *Riverrun* and impressionist music—although Takemitsu's work is the result of this composer's fascination for George Russell's influential jazz book *The Lydian Chromatic Concept of Tonal Organization for Improvisation*. Machart does not answer one important question readers may ponder: does the minimalist aesthetic lend itself to an elegiac affective quality, or is this trait unique to John Adams among all the minimalist composers? The second half of the excerpted book explores music boxes, or the propensity for machine gadgetry in music. Machart believes that Adams's works ranging from 1991 to 1996 are governed by machine-like processes that sometimes end up falling apart like toys. I would concur that in some fashion these works give commentary on minimalism by thwarting musical structures and natural unfolding processes. Machart likens the Chamber Symphony to a robot that spins out of control. The notion of the machine working in Adams's Violin Concerto is accomplished through Adams's signature rising scales during the first movement, which Machart fails to attribute to its mechanized process. The two-piano work *Hallelujah Junction* is compared to Fracis Poulenc's piano style while combined with the deliberate effect of being in and out of sync through patterns repeated in rapid succession to create an echo effect. For Machart the work *Century Rolls* recalls Steve Reich's *Music for 18 Musicians* in its use of textures and of tonalities. The notion of the machine is prominent in this work through the pulsation of a pacemaker beat. Machart's tour of Adams's works concludes with *Slonimsky's Earbox*, which he believes is a kind of experiment for the "swollen" chords and ultra-complex writing of *Naive and Sentimental Music*.

10.   May, Thomas, ed. *The John Adams Reader: Essential Writings on an American Composer.* Pompton Plains: Amadeus, 2006.

In *The John Adams Reader*, Thomas May presents a compilation of articles from both scholarly sources and newspaper articles on a wide range of topics. May's book provides a great deal of background information on John Adams's compositions, and May also devotes a large portion of the book to the critical reception of Adams's works, particularly the controversial nature of his opera *The Death of Klinghoffer*, as some critics have argued the opera endorses anti-Semitism. For the opening chapter, titled "John Adams Reflects on His Career," Thomas May interviewed John Adams in 2005 while the composer was in residence at Northwestern University. May opens with a question about Adams's interest in musical composition at an early age, to which the composer describes his first composition, a minuet. Adams discusses other important musical activities during his early life, such as listening to Bach's Brandenburg Concertos and Mozart on his family's Magnavox long-playing record console. May fast-forwards to musical experiences during the Harvard years, delving into the angst of being a tonal composer during a time in which atonal music was the only acceptable medium of musical expression in academia. Adams recalls his thoughts on the music of Schoenberg and other Second Viennese composers along with the general ambiance about music composition at Harvard at the time, one of longing for the days of tonal music yet being unable to turn away from Schoenberg's dominating influence. Then Adams tells how he came at a crossroads between Pierre Boulez's scientific methods or John Cage's Zen philosophies.

After Harvard, Adams ventures to the West Coast for its musical and literary scene at the time. He reveals his love of Henry Miller's *Big Sur*, which later formed the title for *The Dharma at Big Sur*. Reflecting on his early works, Adams declares the 1973 *American Standard* as the germinating point for his more mature compositions, despite the fact that it lacked the harmonic and rhythmic language of his *Gate* works from the late 70s. Adams talks about his compositional process at length, detailing issues like orchestration, proofreading, his daily routine, and the use of music software (Digital Performer) for composition. He describes his concept of harmonic prolongation or "harmonic flow," which extends harmonies over long arches of time to produce large musical structures. Speaking of the minimalist aesthetic and development, Adams distances himself from the movement for not following its degree of rigidity.

In a subsequent chapter, Thomas May interviews the composer Ingram Marshall regarding his friendship with John Adams. Marshall discusses one of Adams's early pieces, called *Discharging Capacitors*—Adams mentions this early work in his autobiography. *Discharging Capacitors* entails three pieces that utilize small electronic gadgets lying around the floor of a performance hall to make random sounds. The pieces were composed during the mid-70s, during a time Adams was influenced by John Cage's musical aesthetic. Marshall provides specifics on Adams's first encounters with minimalism, meeting Reich, and soon thereafter, performing Reich's *Music for Mallet Instruments, Voices and Organ*. Marshall also gives some information on Adams's master's thesis, a composition titled *Heavy Metal*. Marshall mentions another early work by Adams titled *Studebaker Love Music*.

In a subsequent chapter, May includes a transcript from another interview with the composer during the time Adams was composing *Doctor Atomic*. Speaking on the compositional process, Adams explains he begins writing opera music with just the vocal parts and a very rudimentary piano score, and the orchestration follows last. May and Adams delve into the challenging collaboration with librettist Alice Goodman, which after many disputes, resulted in Goodman abandoning the project. As is known, the libretto for *Doctor Atomic* consists of a compilation of poems, biblical excerpts, and other texts compiled by Adams and Peter Sellars. Adams read numerous books during the planning stage, including but not limited to *The Making of the Atomic Bomb, Dark Star*, and *Bhagavad Gita*, and writings by John Donne. Adams tackles the misnomer that he is a political composer, stating that all life is intertwined with politics. The last topic they touch upon is the state, longevity, and function of opera in today's society.

Next, May interviews Adams's lifelong collaborator Peter Sellars. They discuss Sellars's first encounter with Adams during the early 1980s. Regarding their opera collaborations, Sellars and Adams both believe the "CNN opera" moniker is a mischaracterization of their work. Sellars opines their opera delves deeper than the news medium because it dramatizes the characters' underlying motives. Regarding the portrayal of the East in *Nixon in China*, Sellars reveals that musically speaking the opera has no overt Chinese reference like *The Mikado*, and the deliberate avoidance of orientalism in favor of shared music is what binds the two cultures in the opera. Sellars concludes with *Doctor Atomic*, comparing it with Wagner's *Götterdämmerung*, an opera of epic proportions, for pathos and subject matter. Moreover, both operas explore the end of the world but from different angles: myth and reality.

In "Robert Spano on Conducting the Music of John Adams," May interviews the music director of the Atlanta Symphony to speak on his experiences conducting Adams's works. This conductor is a proponent of Adams's music and of other contemporary composers. Spano discusses overall challenges in conducting Adams's music. Maestro Spano talks in length about the diversity of Adams's musical style and how unique each work feels under the baton. From a conductor's point of view, Spano considers Adams an architectural composer, on par with Bach, Mozart, Sibelius, and Tchaikovsky.

In "Emanuel Ax on Performing Adams's Piano Concerto," May interviews Ax during his tour with fellow pianist Yefim Bronfman in the spring of 2005. As is known, Ax, together with the Cleveland Orchestra, commissioned Adams's piano concerto *Century Rolls*. Ax delves into an interesting array of topics. First, he reflects on how he approached learning Adams's concerto, which is vastly different from the usual classical repertoire he is known for interpreting. Ax recounts that initial performances served as testing ground to determine parts where the piano required greater audibility; thus, microphone amplification of the piano was deemed as one of the workable solutions at the time. Apparently, it seemed satisfactory to Adams, who then added instructions for amplification on the score. Ax describes the style of *Century Rolls* as a combination of romantic sensibilities with a postminimalist style unique to Adams. Ax further opines it is easy to program Adams with works by Bruckner and other great classics—perhaps because of its accessibility as it eschews the notion of only few cognoscenti to grasp the music.

Continuing the book's section on interpreters of Adams's works, May interviews "Dawn Upshaw on Singing in *El Niño*," which took place in March 2005. Although Upshaw had performed and recorded Adams's music before *El Niño*, this more recent work marks her first project she worked with the composer. Adams consulted with Upshaw on the making of the "Memorial de Tlatelolco" scene from *El Niño*, and Upshaw compares it in difficulty to Stravinsky's *The Rake's Progress*, an opera she worked on during her early career. Adams adhered to Upshaw's advice for a short break in the vocal line during the second half of the oratorio. For Upshaw, the term *oratorio* does not capture the essence of this work. She believes there is more development of a story line than in an oratorio; thus, it situates itself somewhere in between opera and oratorio. Upshaw contends that Adams's text setting deliberately accents the natural flow of words, and therefore feels very natural. Even in a late work such as *El Niño*, Upshaw believes the large-scale structure, which unfolds gradually, is the unifying principle of the oratorio, a quality akin to minimalist and postminimalist works.

11.   Müller-Berg, Sandra. *"Tonal Harmony Is Like a Natural Force": Eine Studie über das Orchesterwerk Harmonielehre von John Adams*. Hofheim: Wolke-Verlag, 2006.

Müller-Berg's book derives out of her 2006 dissertation that bears the same title. The author gives an in-depth study of Adams's *Harmonielehre*. The author regards Adams's musical work as a prototypical model for postmodernist music. Following an introduction of the work, the second chapter lists musical influences that take shape in *Harmonielehre*, including Sibelius's Fourth Symphony, Mahler's Fourth and Tenth Symphonies, and Schoenberg's *Gurre-Lieder* and *Erwartung*. In the third chapter, the author examines Schoenberg's theoretical treatise *Harmonielehre* and considers its implications on Adams's work. The following chapter explores Adams's notions of harmony, tonality, and modulation. Additionally, Müller-Berg elaborates on rhythm, harmony, and formal aspects of Adams's *Harmonielehre* and the manner in which these musical parameters can be reasoned through Schoenberg's theories.

12.   Potter, Keith, Kyle Gann, and Pwyll ap Siôn, eds. *The Ashgate Research Companion to Minimalist and Postminimalist Music*. Farnham: Ashgate Publishing Company, 2013.

This book provides the most thorough and recent volume on minimalism and its development over a period of more than fifty years. Its varied range of contributing authors offers a full gamut of topics for the study of minimalism and postminimalism. A number of Adams's works are considered, to the extent possible in such a broad volume that reflects on the entire history of this musical style. In their introduction, the editors aim to encapsulate the primary character- istics of the minimalist style, using terms and musical concepts such as harmonic stasis, repetition, drones, gradual process, steady beat, static instrumentation, metamusic, pure tuning, and audible structure. The authors consider the initial references to the term *postminimalism*—coined by Rockwell to describe John Adams's minimalist/neo-Romantic postmodern music—and seek to explain it as a style that employs repetition to musical layers and textures, but not to the level of structure, as is the case with the former. Yet another defining aspect is its infusion of other musical styles. The editors refer to John Adams as the "fifth minimalist" (succeeding Riley, Young, Glass, and Reich) and assert that his early works incorporate quotation and reference into pattern-based minimalism—the same can be said of various post-*Nixon* works.

Pwyll ap Siôn expands on this subject in his own chapter, "Reference and Quo- tation in Minimalist and Postminimalist Music." Ap Siôn considers quotation as a means of parody in Adams's output from his early period, including *American Standard* and *Grand Pianola Music*. Another important aspect this book traces is the development of minimalism and the distinguishing terms *minimalism* and *postminimalism*.

From a music-theoretical standpoint, Tristian Evans's chapter on analytical meth- odologies for postminimalist music gives a broad survey of the approaches that critical writings have applied, offering a concise "history of music theory" and its development confined to the minimalist style. Evans purports that approaches have shifted in recent writings, moving away from traditional structuralist ana- lytical approaches (such as set theory) towards poststructuralist approaches (such as Nicholas Cook's hermeneutic models for understanding multimedia works). Evans's survey provides a useful (though incomplete) foundation for addressing analytical aspects of John Adams's music. Additional annotations from this book can be searched by each individual author.

13. Ross, Alex. *The Rest Is Noise: Listening to the Twentieth Century*. New York: Farrar, Straus and Giroux, 2007.

Ross presents a fresh survey of twentieth-century music and offers a closer look at its composers. He provides biographical narratives and historical information, including social and cultural aspects, as well as firsthand accounts. Ross has the vantage point of writing and reflecting on musical styles and innovations that stem from a previous century. The author uses eye-catching titles that focus on a range of composers, such as "Beethoven was Wrong: Bop, Rock, and the Min- imalists." Ross's chapter on minimalism compares New York and West Coast styles and their development, and examines the musical symbiosis experienced between jazz, rock 'n' roll, and classical composers. While Adams is discussed in brevity, Ross offers interesting ideas worthy of consideration. Ross hypothesizes that Adams was drawn to the music of Sibelius as an archetypical compositional model. Ross furnishes the historical context of Adams's *Harmonielehre*, as well as a synopsis (along with some relevant commentary) of *Nixon in China*.

14.   Schwarz, K. Robert. *Minimalists*. London: Phaidon, 1996.

K. Robert Schwarz's *Minimalists*, considered a classic, discusses a wide range of minimalist composers, including La Monte Young, Terry Riley, Steve Reich, Philip Glass, John Adams, Meredith Monk, Michael Nyman, Louis Andriessen, and Arvo Pärt. The book highlights the origins of minimalism, stemming as a reaction to Darmstadt avant-garde influences. A significant portion of the book focuses on biographical information, where the author discusses Adams's time as a graduate student at Harvard. Schwarz identifies Adams as the original postminimalist composer whose contribution to the minimalist style infused the simplicity of minimalism with the passion of Romanticism. The author includes Adams's bold claim that minimalism stands as "the only really interesting important stylistic development in the past thirty years." Schwarz introduces some of Adams's less commonly known works, including *American Standard* and *Lo-Fi*. The author epitomizes Adams's *Phrygian Gates* and *Shaker Loops* as musical statements in an eclectic minimalist vocabulary, offering a short overview of each work. Adams views the development of any musical style as originating in the simplest ways and transforming into a more complex language, and to this, minimalism is no exception. Schwarz believes the synthesis of minimalism and Romanticism continues in Adams's *Harmonium* and *Harmonielehre*, and he visits these two works with that perspective. *Grand Pianola Music* shows a shift in style and a way to reclaim the popular culture. This work along with *Fearful Music* and others are often regarded by writers as Adams's "trickster" pieces for their playful, vernacular, and irreverent character. Schwarz forges ahead in Adams's career to explore Adams's *Nixon in China*. There are noteworthy quotations regarding Adams's views on opera repertoire and his desire to break away from those opera subjects "so completely out of touch in this century." Adams discusses his interest in Jungian psychology and the nature of myths and archetypes in operas such as *Nixon in China*. Schwarz compares elements of Glass's music to *Nixon in China* and argues that subsequent to this opera, Adams relies upon the framework of minimalism only as one compositional technique among many, thus distancing himself further from minimalist roots.

4

Journal and Magazine Articles, Book Chapters

15. Ashby, Arved. "Minimalist Opera." In *The Cambridge Companion to Twentieth-Century Opera*, ed. Mervyn Cooke, 244–66. Cambridge: Cambridge University Press, 2005.

Ashby views the genesis of minimalist music as an offshoot of avant-garde New York theater. Philip Glass was one of the pioneers, and his experiences with the Living Theatre and their *Frankenstein* productions had a profound impact on his sense of time in music making. The author notes that before the 1960s, American music and theater were generally not performed in opera houses. In Adams's *Nixon in China*, a work Ashby regards as the culmination of minimalist opera, the medium of video and television appropriate notions of musical theater. For Ashby, *Nixon in China* holds an important role in contemporary operatic literature as the first opera to recognize the operatic value of television. Ashby elaborates on the role of static and dynamic repetition in minimalist music as a reaction of Darmstadt modernism and views it in light of Gilles Deleuze's book *Difference and Repetition*, originally published in French during the time Glass and Reich were developing their minimalist sound. Ashby devotes attention to contrasting operatic and oratorio elements of *The Death of Klinghoffer*, noting Adams's second opera provides a stark contrast to the first. Ashby also weighs in on the controversial nature of Adams's operas, which he believes is contributed by its failing to choose one side of the moral compass, noting that opera, by tradition, chooses sides. On a different note, readers might be cautious to accept Ashby's facile descriptions of Adams's postminimalist style, since Adams experimented in earnest with early minimalism at the beginning of his career. Additionally, I remain puzzled as to why Ashby entertains the idea that Adams's postminimalist style might be construed as opportunistic hypocrisy.

16.   Atkinson, Sean. "Aspects of Otherness in John Adams's *Nixon in China*." *Dutch Journal of Music Theory* 18, no. 3 (2013): 155–69.

Atkinson gives an in-depth examination of *Nixon in China* by considering the music in conjunction with other aspects of the production, focusing on the action on stage. The author investigates the way Adams depicts *otherness*, deliberately avoiding attempts to replicate Chinese music. This means avoiding traditional markers associated with Chinese music, including pentatonicism, high-register instrumentation, and the imitation of eastern folk instruments. Atkinson cites Timothy Johnson's work to illustrate how Adams's harmonic language can be elucidated using principles of neo-Riemannian theory. While Adams's harmonic world is Western in origin, despite the traditional markers that evoke Eastern culture, Atkinson purports that Adams creates a sense of otherness in the opera. The author asserts that Adams's opera provides commentary on other twentieth-century operas that have wrestled with exoticism and otherness—the most famous instance being Puccini's *Madama Butterfly*. Atkinson's analyses respond to Johnson's book *John Adams's Nixon in China: Musical Analysis, Historical and Political Perspectives*. Like Johnson, Atkinson employs transformational theory to elucidate moments when the opera narrative is at odds with the music, which endows the opera and the characters in the opera with a sense of satire and sarcasm. Another area of analysis Atkinson incorporates in his article entails musical semiotics and the study of topics, which highlights how the opera has the capacity to evoke marches, pastoral music, and other musical scenes. In the concluding segment of his article, Atkinson discusses the effects of staging on the meaning of the opera and the notion of otherness. The two most striking changes made by Sellars in the 2011 Metropolitan Opera production affect two important scenes: Madame Mao motions for Ching-hua to shoot Lao Szu, which she finally does in the latter production, as well as the portrayal of Premier Chou's death on stage in the most recent production.

17.   Baier, Christian. "Der Mythos der Aktualität: John Adams' *The Death of Klinghoffer* bei den Wiener Festwochen." *Österreichische Musikzeitschrift* 46, no. 5 (1991): 234–36. In German.

Following the 1991 world premiere of *The Death of Klinghoffer* in Brussels, the opera was subsequently staged later that year at the Vienna Festival. Baier introduces German-speaking readers to Adams's musical influences and style of composition. He purports that the present-day mythology portrayed in Adams's second opera does not rely on allegory (unlike works by Hindemith, Britten, and others) to create a sense of timelessness.

18.   Bauer, Cornelius. "Adams Reloaded: Überlegungen zu John Adams' aktuellem Komponieren anhand von *Son of Chamber Symphony* (2007)." In *Musik, Kultur, Wissenschaft*, eds. Hartmut Möller and Martin Schröder, 81–105. Essen: Verlag Die Blaue Eule, 2011. In German.

Bauer reflects on Adams's mature compositional style, examining *Son of Chamber Symphony* as a model. He introduces the minimalist aesthetic and Adams's compositional style to German readers not acquainted with the subject matter. Bauer notes that Adams's Chamber Symphony exhibited a radical shift from his earlier style in its unparalleled degree of complexity. Subsequent compositions continued Adams's new path towards a contrapuntal language interwoven within the minimalist framework. Bauer includes analysis of Adams's *Son of Chamber Symphony* with musical illustrations, touching on musical form, harmony, and motivic and phrase analysis. The author characterizes the second movement as less complex, comprising a lyrical melody over a chordal accompaniment. The third movement resembles a rondo form. The author opines that Adams still operates on a harmonic palette consisting of triads and seventh chords, though expressed linearly. His harmonic analysis tracks changes in pitch center and diatonic mode. Bauer purports the opening measures of Adams's symphony are a direct quotation from Beethoven's Symphony No. 9. The author also notes Adams's minimalist tendencies and tracks how repeated patterns transform over time, as well as how free melodies come into the fore and gradually morph into ostinato figures. Overall, this article presents a good introduction to Adams's *Son of Chamber Symphony*.

19. Beckwith, John. "Anhalt's *Oppenheimer*: The History of a Never-Finished Work." *Intersections: Canadian Journal of Music/Revue canadienne de musique* 33, no. 2 (2013): 101–14.

Beckwith discusses Istvan Anhalt's unfinished opera on the same subject as Adams's *Doctor Atomic*. The author compares the work from both of these composers. The libretto envisioned by Anhalt and his librettist Murrell covers a thirty-year segment of Oppenheimer's life, while Adams and Sellar's libretto focuses on the events in 1945. Furthermore, Beckwith elaborates on differences of text used in each of the operas. The findings appear to be overly concise for detailed study, though Beckwith points the reader to an unpublished study by musicologist Peter Laki that compares the two operas at length (see item 59).

20. Beirens, Maarten. "Het culturele slachtoffer van 11 september: De controverse rond John Adams." *Contra. Stemmen over muziek* 2, no. 3 (2002): 20–23. In Dutch.

Beirens discusses Adams's controversial reputation as the composer of *The Death of Klinghoffer*, siding with Adams against Taruskin's attacks on alleged grounds of anti-Semitism. Beirens also explores Adams's newest work at the time, *On the Transmigration of Souls*.

21. Bernard, Jonathan W. "Minimalism, Postminimalism, and the Resurgence of Tonality in Recent American Music." *American Music* 21, no. 1 (2003): 112–33.

This article helps classify contemporary composers' works who employ extensive repetition in their music into three categories: minimalist, postminimalist, or neither. Bernard describes four criteria in the development of the minimalist style: (1) minimal pieces gained complexity, (2) a greater concern with sonorities arose, (3) textures became explicitly harmonic, and (4) harmonies of a quasi-tonal essence came to the fore. Bernard states that Adams embraced minimalist traits about ten years after Reich and Glass; for that reason, his music fits into stages three and four. Bernard includes score illustrations of Adams's *Phrygian Gates*, *Fearful Symmetries*, and the Violin Concerto to elucidate Adams's approach to rhythm, pulsation, and its development throughout the composer's career.

22.   Blim, Dan. "'Meaningful Adjacencies': Disunity and the Commemoration of 9/11 in John Adams's *On the Transmigration of Souls.*" *Journal of the Society for American Music* 7, no. 4 (2013): 382–420.

Blim presents a musicological study of Adams's *On the Transmigration of Souls*, working with the premise that the role of disunity serves the process of memorializing the 9/11 tragedy. Blim's approach gathers studies from musical and cultural analysis with concert audience surveys conducted in six cities between 2010 and 2012. The survey reproduced in Appendix A asks audience members to rate the various affective qualities they perceive, record any images the work conjures in their mind, and reflect on the underlying message Adams's music expresses. Furthermore, Blim's article incorporates various audience members' impressions of the musical by borrowing their emotive descriptors. By incorporating audience responses, Blim posits that disunity between and within music and text evokes the experience of traumatic memories, acknowledges absence, and enables the composer and listener to "navigate among multiple competing identities, particularly for those citizens who did not fit the dominant narrative of white male heroism following 9/11 (384). The dichotomy of presence and absence are at the foreground of Blim's investigation. Another important theme explored is the relationship between minimalism and memorial spaces. Using a waveform graph of the entire work, the author highlights the structure of Adams's work, showing how the two climaxes represent the destruction of the two towers. Blim offers a musical synopsis of Adams's commemorative work, addressing instrumental forces and musical climaxes that work in tandem with a second orchestral group performing a quarter-tone higher, a compositional technique influenced by Charles Ives. Blim proves further, comparing thematic ideas from Ives's *The Unanswered Question* and Aaron Copland's *Quiet City* and asserting that Adams's work resists closure by blurring boundaries between music and sound.

23.   Buch, Esteban. "Musique, mémoire et critique du 11 Septembre: à propos de *On The Transmigration of Souls* de John Adams." In *Faire des sciences sociales: critiquer*, eds. Pascale Haag and Cyril Lemieux, 289–316. Paris: Editions de l'EHESS, 2012. In French.

Buch examines the political discourse created by Adams's *On the Transmigration of Souls* in remembering 9/11. Buch contrasts Adams's work with Bruce Springsteen's 2001 song *The Rising*, written to honor the heroism of the 9/11 firefighters. Whereas Springsteen's song affirms the outrage and group solidarity in the United States, Adams's work is characterized by what Hervé Guibert calls a compassion protocol. The work aids in creating this ambiance through modality, homophony, and sounds that evoke the feeling of a cathedral. Adams's collected sources from the victims create a mosaic, but one that omits references to God or Islam, perhaps in attempts to reach a broad audience under the umbrella of the American collective. Buch disagrees with other scholars' assertion that the work's bipartite formal construction mirrors the twin towers because of their apparent musical asymmetry. Buch devotes attention to sorting out critics' impressions of these works, noting that the response from Terry Teachout that Adams's work does not express faith, love, or hope, but rather uncertainty. While Buch does not subscribe to Teachout's point of view, he opines that Adams's work is positioned too close to conventions and too far from critique to offer an alternative perspective on the memory of the terrorist attack.

24.   Cahill, Sarah. "Performance Anxiety and Minimalism." In *The Ashgate Research Companion to Minimalist and Postminimalist Music*, eds. Keith Potter, Kyle Gann, and Pwyll Ap Siôn, 385–7. Farnham: Ashgate Publishing Limited, 2013.

Pianist Cahill speaks about the challenges and anxiety of performing minimalist piano repertoire. She elaborates on Adams's piano piece *China Gates*, which the composer dedicated to her in 1977. Cahill references Terry Riley's *Keyboard Studies*, which, according to her description of interlocking patterns of differing lengths in each hand, resemble the same kind of technique found in the middle section of *China Gates*. During a performance of minimalist repertoire, she remarks, it is more difficult to recover after a mistake than in classical repertoires. Cahill notes that while she has performed *China Gates* for thirty-five years, during a recent performance she lost her focus and was unable to find her place on the score due to the visual homogeneity of the formal sections. Cahill believes performance practices of minimalist repertoire have evolved during their brief existence. While Adams himself included performance instructions advising pianists to play at a soft dynamic level and to refrain from accenting patterns and individual notes, Cahill informs readers that Adams today views performance practices more freely. Pianists now are encouraged to interpret the gate pieces by considering the interaction between melodic lines, the tension between modes, and the use of the sustain pedal, and even playing louder than mezzo-forte. The subject of performance practices of other musical styles has been discussed, most notably by Richard Taruskin in *Text and Act: Essays on Music and Performance*, and the same arguments of performing historically or, on the other side of the spectrum, in a presentist mode, come to the fore in Adams's minimalist piano pieces. One of the main points in Cahill's chapter delves into how listeners' apprehensions towards minimalist pieces have changed over time, which has shaped the status of *China Gates* into one of the staples in the minimalist vein.

25.   Carl, Robert. "Six Case Studies in New American Music: A Postmodern Portrait Gallery." *College Music Symposium* 30, no. 1 (1990): 45–63.

Carl's article is a sequel to his 1989 "The Politics of Definition in New Music," which highlights the struggle between postmodernism and minimalism. In his current article, Carl asserts that composers like Adams have achieved a synthesis between the two aesthetic aims described in his earlier article. Carl, like

other authors, purports that Adams is the most successful contemporary concert composer. The author refers to Adams as a second-generation minimalist
and a crossover minimalist who skirts between minimalism and mainstream
influences. Carl describes Adams's early pieces as a metamorphosis of harmony
and color. The author believes that Adams owes his success to his experiences as
composer-in-residence with the San Francisco Symphony, where the composer
became more attuned to musical tastes of audience members. Adams's infusion
of romantic and minimalist styles surfaces in works from *Harmonium* onwards
for their quicker changes of harmonic progression. Carl believes *Harmonielehre*
and *Grand Pianola Music* suffer from being kitschy and not memorable or imag-
inative. This minor quibble does not affect the way Carl views *Nixon in China*
and *Short Ride in a Fast Machine* as having achieved a real synthesis of romantic
and minimalist aesthetic elements. Overall, Carl's assessment of Adams's growth
(up to the year 1990) is a positive one, and he even likens Adams's appropriation
of popular and vernacular styles to Aaron Copland.

26.   Cervo, Dimitri. "Post-Minimalism: Is It a Valid Terminology?" *Ictus* 1 (1999):
       37–52.

Cervo describes postminimalist music as a stylistic shift away from early minimalist works. According to the author, Robert Pincus-Witten coined the term
postminimalism to describe a period of American art between 1966 and 1976
that sought to eschew the aesthetic of impersonality brought on by early minimalism. Cervo contends that the principal distinction between early and late
representations of the minimalist style regards early minimalism as a byproduct
of modernism, imbued with radical, systematic, and exclusionist traits. He argues
that the term *postminimalism* can be justified only if it can be recognized in a
sizable corpus of music by numerous composers, and postulates that postminimalist works share three main features: (1) stylistic eclecticism, (2) the incorporation of foregrounded melodic lines, and (3) the presence of multi-movements
or sections within a single work. Cervo then cites statements by Reich and Glass
that corroborate their attempts to loosen the strictures of the style. The author
remarks that Adams's attempt to wean from early minimalist aesthetic came in
the form of dramatic musical works.

27.   Christiansen, Rupert. "Breaking Taboos (Portrait of Alice Goodman)." *Opera*
       (May 2003). Reprinted in *The John Adams Reader: Essential Writings on an
       American Composer*, ed. Thomas May, 249–57. Pompton Plains: Amadeus, 2006.

Christiansen introduces and gives commentary on Alice Goodman's libretti from
Nixon in China and *The Death of Klinghoffer*. He explores Goodman's difficult
relationship with Adams and reiterates Goodman's opinion that "the librettist is
rather more than a servant to the composer" (250). Goodman's harsh criticism of
Adams's earlier works set the tone for their pre-arranged collaboration. Her first
impressions of Adams's *Harmonium*—"What has [Adams] done to Dickinson's
and Donne's words?"—reveals her judgmental tone over an art form foreign to

her own creative process. The collaboration for *The Death of Klinghoffer* was even rockier than *Nixon* because choreographer Mark Morris was added to the equation. Christiansen cites Goodman's recollections of the events that led to the *Klinghoffer* controversy, a public outcry that the opera glamorized terrorist Palestinian ideologies. Naturally, Goodman disagrees with Richard Taruskin's condemnation of her libretto and feels people reacted strongly because the libretto violates certain taboos. Goodman adheres to the Elizabethan line of thought where both sides of a story are presented with neutrality, just as Shakespeare does in *Macbeth* or *Coriolanus*.

28.   Conway, Eoin. "Signature Characteristics in the Piano Music of John Adams." *Maynooth Musicology* 2 (2009): 220–35.

Conway investigates musical factors that allow listeners to instantaneously recognize Adams's music upon first hearing. Conway's study focuses on texture, melody, rhythm, and harmony in Adams's piano works. In the areas of texture and melody, Conway describes Adams's earliest minimalist technique as juxtaposed melodies built from scale fragments or arpeggios. To provide greater contrast and avoid some literal repetition in *China Gates* and *Phrygian Gates*, Adams's repeated textures contain opposing lengths. Textures are punctuated by sporadic notes entering at irregular intervals in a higher register than juxtaposed patterns. These two techniques occur on a grand scale in *Common Tones in Simple Time*, *Harmonium*, and *Grand Pianola Music*. Later in the 1980s Adams developed a penchant for oscillating harmonies. Conway uses the term *oscillating note motif* to describe how multiple individual oscillations contribute to melodic content in Adams's works for piano, such as *Hallelujah Junction*. Conway asserts that Adams's rhythms for piano are percussive in nature and fall under several categories: a stride piano adapted for the composer's minimalist idiom, rhythms of interlocking patterns reminiscent of medieval hocket, and ostinato patterns shared between the hands, such as those from *Road Movies*. Subsequent to *Nixon in China*, *Eros Piano* transforms triadic structures into harmonies of superimposed fifths. Conway notes that the opening of *Eros Piano* stems from a quote from the end of Takemitsu's *Riverrun*. According to the author, majorseventh chords assume a structural role in *Eros Piano* (the same may be said of *Road Movies* and *Century Rolls*). The author posits that *Eros Piano* marks the end of Adams's first compositional period of writing for piano solo or within an ensemble. Adams's use of polyharmony in *Road Movies* signals a new trend in Adams's stylistic order. This technique emanates during moments of aggression or conflict, such as in scenes from *The Death of Klinghoffer* that portray anger or malice. Other works in this vein include *Hallelujah Junction* and *American Berserk*. Another important sonority, the minor-seventh chord, is mentioned in reference to works such as *Lollapalooza* and *Century Rolls* and described as distinctively Adamsian. Overall, Conway provides an important inventory of signature techniques that contribute to Adams's style, which expands ideas from Dan Warburton's 1988 "A Working Terminology for Minimal Music."

29.   Cook, Karen M. "Music, History, and Progress in Sid Meier's *Civilization IV*." In *Music in Video Games: Studying Play*, eds. K. J. Donnelly, William Gibbons, and Neil Lerner, 166–82. New York: Routledge, 2014.

Cook writes a study on the young field of ludomusicology, or the study of music in video games. Cook identifies nine works from Adams's oeuvre contained in the 2005 video game *Civilization 4*, centered on building on a macro-scale throughout different eras: Medieval, Renaissance, Industrial, and Modern. Cook affirms that the Modern era is exclusively represented using Adams's compositions that she catalogs in her study, including *Christian Zeal and Activity, Common Tones in Simple Time, Grand Pianola Music, Shaker Loops, Harmonielehre, The Chairman Dances, Tromba Lontana, Nixon in China*, and the Violin Concerto. Cook opines that Adams's minimalist compositions, which differ vastly from composers chosen for other eras of the game, provide a musical narrative that matches the technologies of the Modern era. Cook considers the implications of representing earlier ears with a wide array of composers versus scoring the Modern era entirely with Adams's works. Concerning the process of importing Adams's works into a musical game in a unified manner, Cook references an interview with Soren Johnson, lead designer for *Civ IV*, who believes Adams's works have the right kind of forward momentum for the game. For practical purposes, Johnson maintains it was necessary to remove certain portions from Adams's works that were climatic and overly dissonant.

30.   Daines, Matthew. "Nixon's Women: Gender Politics and Cultural Representation in Act 2 of *Nixon in China*." *The Musical Quarterly* 79, no. 1 (1995): 6–34.

This contribution to the area of opera and gender studies examines the roles portrayed by the principal characters of *Nixon in China*. Daines targets the following themes in his study: Pat Nixon as a historical character, Pat Nixon as an operatic character, Madame Mao as a historical character, the historical version of the Red Detachment of Women, and the reincarnation of the Red Detachment of Women in Nixon in China. According to Daines, gender issues play a critical role in Adams's opera. The first act introduces the male characters, the second introduces the female characters, and the third act features the principal male and female characters in a mode of self-reflection as they contemplate their lives.

As a historical figure, Pat Nixon is viewed as having a stoic and even repressed personality, in contrast with the operatic character in the opera. As an opera character, Pat plays a remarkable role in the relations between both countries with her strength of character. The music Adams sets for Pat Nixon showcases a compositional technique Daines describes as intercutting the libretto, where a chorus sung by her Chinese hosts is interwoven in arias such as "I don't daydream." Daines describes the function of the chorus as a way to form a bond to Pat Nixon and vocalize her feelings of loneliness. In Daines's reading of the opera, Pat Nixon plays an equal role to Richard Nixon. She takes excursions to visit sites and see people, speaks of American and Chinese values, and even ponders on the meaning of world peace. Adams and Goodman make an effort to reflect on her private persona more than her public image.

Mao Tse-tung's fourth and final wife, Chiang Ch'ing, presents an opposite end of the spectrum from Pat Nixon. She ranked third after Chairman Mao and Chou En-lai. She was conceivably the most powerful woman in the world. In the opera, Ch'ing is depicted as abrasive and aggressive, which mirrors the harsh life she had led. The final portion of the article discusses gender issues outside of the opera, including Goodman's collaboration with Adams and Sellars and published criticism of the opera, mostly reviewed by men. In support of Daines's examination of Adams's opera, *The Cambridge Companion to Opera Studies*, published in 2012 and edited by Nicholas Till, contains scholarship that is more current on opera and gender studies.

31. _____. "Opera and Layers of Meaning: Act III of *Nixon in China*." *The Opera Journal* 27, no. 4 (1994): 2–13.

Daines detects that early reception of Adams's first opera has been lukewarm, due primarily to critics focusing their attention on the first act, which presents a snapshot of the Nixons' diplomatic trip to China. The third act is largely ignored by critics; however, Daines asserts that it is the most concentrated act from a musical, dramatic, and psychological perspective. The third act eschews numerous traditions of grand opera; namely, *Nixon* portrays the life of living figures. Moreover, notions of formal musical structure and narrative plot unfold in an unconventional operatic fashion. Psychologically, in the third act, we witness the interaction of male and female characters: Chairman Mao dances with Chiang Ch'ing (the well-known scene *The Chairman Dances* occurs here), and the Nixons privately reflect on their marriage and their past. Musically, Adams portrays these interchanges intimately through more contrapuntal textures that interweave and interlock with the voices. As Adams has stated, the musical setting from the third act shows a stark contrast to the homophonic writing in the first two acts. Daines purports the final act focuses on what the characters share in common—their humanity—and musically Adams blurs their personalities. Every character in this act partakes in a series of duets and trios. Another distinction between the first two acts and the final one is evident, due to the personal nature of this act: Peter Sellars's restaging of the original banquet scene is eventually replaced by six beds that resemble coffins. Another interesting observation Daines notes is that the recapitulation of musical themes in the third act reflects the characters' recollections of their past selves.

32. Derfler, Brandon. "Two *Harmonielehren*: Schoenberg and John Adams." *GAMUT: Journal of the Georgia Association of Music Theorists* 9 (1999): 17–42.

The author elaborates on musical parallels between Schoenberg and Adams. Derfler's article presents an abridged and revised version of his 1998 master's thesis. Derfler's musical examples and subheadings are also drawn directly from his thesis. The introduction and conclusion are reworked to fit the format of the brief article and to make a case for the direct influence of Schoenberg's works and writings on Adams's *Harmonielehre*.

33.   Duplay, Mathieu. " 'I Speak According to the Book': écriture et logos dans Nixon in China de John Adams et Alice Goodman." *Transatlantica* 1 (2013): 1–19. In French.

Duplay correlates Goodman's style of writing librettos to a longstanding tradition dominated by Ezra Pound, and Adams's compositional innovations to the influence of John Cage. Duplay attempts to describe Nixon's encounter with Maoist China using theories from philosopher Marshall McLuhan's 1964 work *Understanding Media*.

34.   _____. " 'Next Year in Strength and Justice': Oratorio et élégie dans l'oeuvre de John Adams." *Revue Musicorum* 15 (2016): 115–28. In French.

Duplay's study entails an exploration of Adams's oratorios *El Niño* and *The Gospel According to the Other Mary*. Duplay contends that Adams's oratorios present themselves less as a genre or corpus than as a mode of expression and trope on musical elegies. Duplay remarks that even in his earlier works, Adams bears strong affinities to elegiac qualities that link his music to the past and to the spirit of the oratorio.

35.   Everett, Yayoi Uno. " 'Counting Down' Time: Musical Topics in John Adams' *Doctor Atomic*." In *Music Semiotics: A Network of Significations*, ed. Esti Sheinberg, 263–74. Surrey: Ashgate Publishing, 2012.

Everett utilizes music semiotics to examine intertextual aspects of John Adams's music in *Doctor Atomic*. According to Everett, Adams introduces a number of semiotic topics in novel ways that give meaning to the music and tie in with musical styles from previous composers. Her main argument is that semiotic topics contribute to the ontological passing of time, whereas quotation of other musical styles represents the "psychological realm of the subjects who await the countdown" of the atom bomb (264).

36.   Feuchtner, Bernd. "The *Klinghoffer* Debate." In *Opernwelt Jahrbuch*. Seelze: Erhard Friedrich Verlag, 2004. In German. Translated by Thomas May in *The John Adams Reader: Essential Writings on an American Composer*, 299–312. Pompton Plains: Amadeus, 2006.

Feuchtner explores the question of whether *The Death of Klinghoffer* is an anti-Semitic opera by tracing some of its proponents and detractors. This contemporary opera has sparked more controversy in our time than any other, and it remains as controversial today as it was during its premiere in 1991. Over the years, numerous opera houses have refused to stage the opera or withdrawn it from their program due to outside pressure coming from critics, protesters, and prominent figures including politicians and radio personalities. According to Feuchtner, events in recent American history, including the Gulf War and the attacks on September 11, have affected the perceived intentions of the composer in his quest to portray an opera about a tragic event that led to the death of Leon Klinghoffer.

37.   Fink, Robert. "Going with the Flow: Minimalism as Cultural Practice in Post-War America." In *The Ashgate Research Companion to Minimalist and Post-Minimalist Music*, eds. Keith Potter, Kyle Gann, and Pwyll ap Siôn, 201–18. Farnham: Ashgate Publishing Limited, 2013.

Fink aims to elucidate the origins of minimalism by exploring the cultural aspects of American society during the 1960s. Fink asserts that the gaining popularity of radio and television programs, so accustomed to commercial interruptions, gave way to a kind of music where interruption is a basic ingredient. What Fink means by a musical interruption is not the stopping of music but rather the repeating of a musical segment that forces it to loop back in short spurts, thereby interrupting itself. According to Fink, the rise of the television remote control gave way to more unpredictable television programming, which in turn acclimated audiences to experience more complex minimalist music, leading to the advent of the postminimalist style. Fink delves into Adams's works from his early compositional period, starting with the gate works from the late 1970s. For the author, the sudden change of a gate is akin to the changing of a television channel, where the new channel can be unpredictable. Fink asserts that Adams's unpredictable musical processes help define his unique musical style and equate predictable music with the uninteresting. To support this notion, Fink cites Adams on the opening measures of *Nixon in China*: "You never know when the bass is going to change, how tightly the slower scales will be lapped, when the trombone sputters or the 'ding' will appear" (213). Similarly for Fink, Adams's 1992 Chamber Symphony is a "perfect representation of the turbulent television environment of 1992" (214). The viewer flips channels much like the music features metrical conflict along with irregular and disjunct rhythms. Adams's own account purports Fink's assertion: the composer was studying Schoenberg's Chamber Symphony while hearing cartoons across the room, and all of this infused into a great musical Picasso. The cultural influence on Adams's *Harmonielehre* is related to, but different from, the frequent channel surfing from television audiences. Viewers were free to watch commercials, but they would often change channels to avoid them. Television networks were devising new ways to capture audiences by offering short commercials organized more freely. The logic of interruption is replaced by commercial-free interruptions, and thus *Harmonielehre* is regarded as a cinematic symphony drama.

38.   ____. "*Klinghoffer* in Brooklyn Heights." *Cambridge Opera Journal* 17, no. 2 (2005): 173–213.

Fink presents one of the most comprehensive studies on anti-Semitism in Adams's *The Death of Klinghoffer*. The author provides a list of articles—written from the time the opera was published to 2003—on the critical reception of the opera. Fink notes that Adams took pride in portraying the events of the hijacking with neutrality. Fink claims that in order to depict both sides equally, Arabs were illustrated as killers in the conflict but also as human beings. The article serves as a response to Richard Taruskin's condemnation of the opera. In his conclusion, Fink sides with the composer, asserting the opera does not romanticize terror, but rather presents Leon and Marilyn Klinghoffer as an ordinary couple who were the victims of a terrorist act.

39.   Fyr, Kyle. "At 40, Year of the 'Signature Work': The Cases of Cage, Reich and Adams." *Malaysian Music Journal* 6, no. 1 (2017): 1–13.

Fyr highlights the significance of works by Cage (*4'33"*), Reich (*Music for Eighteen Musicians*) and Adams (*Nixon in China*) as landmarks in contemporary American music. For each of these composers, Fyr details the making of their work and investigates their relevance and impact in their compositional development. Fyr cites studies from psychology that support the belief that a person's artistic achievements often occur by the age of forty. The author lists five conditions to meet the criteria of a signature work: in short, they entail works that have a lasting influence on audiences, culture, and even on the composer's subsequent works. The author draws similarities between Cage, Reich, and Adams by asserting that they each had achieved the apex of their development by the age of forty. Fyr strives to find some connection between the composers, and to this aim, he cites Adams's own words on these two earlier composers. In Adams's developmental stage of his career, Cage and Reich served as models worthy of admiration (philosophical in the former and compositional in the latter). Fyr recreates part of Adams's compositional trajectory leading up to the completion of *Nixon in China* at the age of forty. The author cites Alex Ross, who states that *Harmonium* broke a barrier by proving that minimalist techniques could be absorbed into classical forms. *Harmonium* and *Harmonielehre* proved to be a suitable testing ground that culminates with *Nixon in China*. Fyr touches on numerous issues related to *Nixon in China*, including its creation, political subjects in the opera, and musical style. These developments were spurred by a successful composition prior; furthermore, *Nixon in China* marks a turning point that led to further stylistic development as witnessed in Adams's second opera and beyond.

40.   Germano, William. "Opera as News: *Nixon in China* and the Contemporary Operatic Subject." *University of Toronto Quarterly* 81, no. 4 (2012): 805–23.

Germano regards *Nixon in China* to be one of the first operas written about a factual contemporary subject. The author agrees with Adams that the opera is difficult to categorize. While numerous writers consider *Nixon in China* to be a political opera, Germano posits it is political in nature only to the extent that it features a contemporary political event. Regarding the role of opera as a historical document, Germano cites Herbert Lindenberger's studies on the subject. According to this referenced author, opera is incapable of rendering the past in linguistic terms; instead, its role is to reflect on crises of feeling from those historical events. Other writers are also cited to support the idea that historical figures transform into mythical figures in the operatic stage. After untangling how historical topics function in opera, Germano organizes his subsequent discussion into three topics: telling time in opera, *Nixon* as operatic history, and history as mystery. Contrary to a historical relating of *Nixon*'s events, the operatic medium projects time in multiple ways, through the juxtaposition of the audience experiencing time, the musical delivery, and the plasticity of the work itself. As Germano explores the historical Nixon and the collaboration between Adams and the librettist Goodman, he posits that historical and archival evidence is inseparable from the political imagining of the creators of the opera. Goodman's libretto harkens back to nineteenth-century operas in its verse structure, situating the contemporary subject in an earlier musical period. Contemporary mythology in *Nixon* is experienced in its reference to America's space program, which, according to Germano, resonates the dream of individual discovery and boundlessness and reinvents the idea of an empire. Additionally, and towards the end of the opera, Mao refers to mythology's eternal charm. Germano sums up his article with a statement that in the medium of opera, history becomes crisis and response, action and mythology.

41.   Goehr, Lydia. "The Musicality of Violence: On the Art and Politics of Displacement." In *Elective Affinities: Musical Essays on the History of Aesthetic Theory*, 171–203. New York: Columbia University Press, 2008.

Goehr explores musical works written in commemoration, mourning, or resistance of social and political violence. The author shows a keen interest in the stance that composers adopt toward the victims of violent acts. Goehr elaborates on murder as fine art and censorship in music, supporting her ideas with writings ranging from the ancient Greeks to Adorno and Nietzsche. There are a number of musical works considered: an oratorio by Tippett, two late works by Schoenberg, and Adams's *The Death of Klinghoffer*. Goehr brings up a novel idea to the argument on whether or not Adams's opera is anti-Semitic, stating an Aristotelian fear that audiences will interrupt the opera if not made aware of fact versus fiction. Furthermore, the distance between the musical work and the audience must be established to regard the recounting of the events as art. Goehr remarks that Giacomo Meyerbeer's *Les Hugenots* is a likely precedent to Adams's inclusion of competing choruses in the opera. Goehr offers criticism of Adams's statement that the opera's message is universal; for this author, the opera ends in a state of ambiguity. Later in the chapter, Goehr comes to terms with what she believes is the work's universal message: that people should move past individual suffering toward recognition of our shared existence.

42.   Hardie, Alistair. "Musical Borrowing as Incarnation: A Theological Reading of Hildegard's *O quam preciosa* in John Adams's *El Niño*." *Contemporary Music Review* 29, no. 3 (2010): 291–307.

Hardie explores how incarnation can be interpreted within a musical narrative in the birth scene of Adams's *El Niño*. The author's opening discourse explains the interconnectivity between music and theology and draws on Jeremy Begbie's *Theology, Music and Time*, published in 2000. The author elaborates on theories of universal time and musical time, noting their interaction between these two temporalities. Hardie analyzes the formal structure from the birth scene, asserting it contains three individual sections connected with transitions and ending with a coda. The sections are delineated by Hildegard's responsory as well as different pitch centers. The author musically interprets God's incarnation in a musical narrative comprising five stages. The first stage presents a conflict between minimalist techniques, which articulate musical form and musical time, with musical material that serves to destabilize the pitch center and rhythm. An unusual nine-note scale, independent of the pervading tonality and rhythm, is representative of God's transcendence. In the second stage, another form of God's transcendence appears in the form of a transposed version of Hildegard's chant, *O quam preciosa*. The author posits that as God is both transcendent and immanent, Hildegard's chant is juxtaposed with earlier musical material resulting in a clash between tonalities. In the third stage, the transposed chant is contrasted with the original chant using the foreground pitch center; the author interprets this musical process as the transcendent chant becoming immanent within the music's content during a transitional stage of the birth scene. The fourth mode entails the synthesis between the two versions of the chant, producing the same nine-note scale, corresponding with text that explicitly portrays the incarnation of Christ. In the fifth stage, transcendent and immanent material is synthesized in musical time, and Hardie concludes that God's transcendence and immanence are similarly joined through Christ's incarnation in universal time. The author opines that Adams intended to explore his own religious beliefs in making *El Niño*. In this regard, his methodological approach seems apt given the subject matter.

43.   Heisinger, Brent. "American Minimalism in the 1980s." *American Music* 7, no. 4 (1989): 430–47.

Heisinger discusses the development of minimalism since its inception to its more recent form in the 1980s. He groups 80s minimalists into four categories: (1) prominent composers whose complete output is minimalist, such as Glass and Reich; (2) composers who occasionally use minimalist techniques, such as Lentz and Rzewski; (3) those who incorporate minimalist techniques in dramatic settings, namely Adams; and (4) composers interested in Indian performance practices, such as Young and Riley. Heisinger characterizes Adams's music from the 80s as having a penchant for diatonicism, repeated cells projecting a sense of pulsation, and a slow harmonic rhythm. Heisinger notes how Adams's music presents yet another departure from early minimalism in how its pulsating figures are often secondary to other musical parameters. Heisinger delves into a broad analysis of minimalist traits in Adams's *Harmonium* while illustrating a score excerpt to highlight his compositional style. The author attributes what he perceives as a goal-oriented quality in Adams's music directly to his sense of drama.

44.   Herzfeld, Gregor. "Tod und Trauer als Narrative neuer Musik: Erinnerungsmusik von Charles Ives, Morton Feldman und John Adams." In *Musik und Narration:*

Philosophische und musikästhetische Perspektiven, eds. Frédéric Döhl and Daniel Martin Feige, 163–91. Bielefeld: Transcript Verlag, 2015. In German.

Herzfeld explores death and grief as a narrative in works by Ives, Feldman, and Adams. The author proposes that in *On the Transmigration of Souls*, Adams depersonalizes subjective grief to facilitate an intermingling of collective and personal mourning. Herzfeld observes that Adams found the notion of a narrative—concerning the plot and consequences—distasteful for the subject matter. However, even if there is no narrative in the strict sense, the narrative content expressed as a temporal structure of musical characters, which are not simply self-referential, but rather tied to musical processes, cannot be overlooked. Herzfeld then interprets the image of millions of pieces of paper fluttering in the sky as a symbol of the victims and their memory, and its density and movement serves as an analog of musical structure. Moreover, the musical layers in conjunction with recorded sounds of the city and the calling of missing persons serve to heighten the consciousness of collective death and grief.

45.   Hill, Andy. "Feed Your Head: Don Davis's *The Matrix.*" In *Scoring the Screen: The Secret Language of Film Music*, 160–94. Milwaukee: Hal Leonard, 2017.

Hill's *Scoring the Screen* explores works of contemporary film composers. In Chapter 7, entitled "Feed Your Head: Don Davis's *The Matrix*," Hill investigates the film score and its musical influence stemming from minimalism, notably, Adams's earlier orchestral works. Hill opines Adams and Davis share a common thread in their manner of creating music through a fabric of repeating cells and large architectonic shapes. Hill relates Davis's compositional use of polyharmony to Adams's *Harmonielehre*, and other works, and purports that conflicting harmonies are suggestive of the protagonist's two worlds presented by the red and blue pills. Hill elaborates on Adams's *gating* technique that dates back to the early piano pieces, and he illustrates a model excerpt from Adams's *Short Ride in a Fast Machine*. Furthermore, Hill asserts that Adams's technique bears a direct applicability to Davis's film score, showing an instance where Trinity, the primary female protagonist, jumps across buildings to defy space and time, while Davis's music undergoes the same kind of *gating* transformation. Subsequently in his book, Hill discusses Adams occasionally, and in relation to his modal and triadic style of writing.

46.   Jankowitz, Christo and Mary Rörich. "What Quackie Said to Meister Eckhart: Intertextuality, Projected Motion and Double-Coding in John Adams's *Harmonielehre.*" *South African Journal of Musicology* 25, no. 1 (2005) 15–29.

Jankowitz and Rörich postulate that compositional periods originate as a form of reaction to the past. A composer's anxiety of influence is expressed in their commentary on music of the past, sometimes through direct or indirect musical quotation, and as a way of atoning preceding traditions. To understand a composer's dialogue with the past through musical texts, styles, or other contextual links, the authors consider the notion of intertextuality. The authors note that

Adams's style is always intertextual but in an eclectic manner that pays homage to the past without the necessity to fully synthesize quotations into a single style. The authors elaborate on Adams's penchant for using the late Romantic sound as a source for inspiration. Their article continues by examining the intertextual surfaces of *Harmonielehre*. Key features of Adams's work are discussed in connections to post-Romantic works. The authors provide citations to assert that Adams's *Harmonielehre* is permeated by double-coding, a strategy of affirming and rejecting existing musical styles. The authors purport that Adams highlights the expressive nature of tonal music while simultaneously parodying the anti-expressive minimalist aesthetic. With this thesis in mind, Jankowitz and Rörich provide a semantic narrative to *Harmonielehre*, portraying the first movement as minimalist in character, the second as being more lyrical, akin to a tonal trope, and the third as fusing minimalist textures with programmatic ideas—Meister Eckhart and Quackie flying through the universe. The authors elaborate on how Adams's second movement pushes late nineteenth-century semiotic buttons and also shows echoes of Shostakovich's Fifth Symphony and Mahler's Tenth Symphony. Another significant allusion to former masterworks is a reference of the "magic sleep" *leitmotif* from Wagner's *Die Walküre*. In their final analysis of *Harmonielehre*, the authors portray Adams as longing for the nineteenth-century sensibilities and thus creating a Romantic simulation unable to match fin-de-siècle drama and tragedy. Furthermore, Jankowitz and Rörich regard Adams's parody in *Harmonielehre* as a commentary on minimalism and not romanticism, an assertion that might seem incongruous with Adams's adoption and development of his postminimalist style.

47.   Johnson, Timothy A. "Harmonic Vocabulary in the Music of John Adams: A Hierarchical Approach." *Journal of Music Theory* 37, no. 1 (1993): 117–56.

The groundwork for this article stems from Johnson's 1991 dissertation. Johnson presents a focused study of Adams's harmonic vocabulary, providing analyses of the composer's works from the 1970s and 80s, including *Phrygian Gates, Harmonium, Harmonielehre,* and *The Chairman Dances.* Johnson updates some of the illustrations presented in his dissertation, including the diagram of the diatonic and superdiatonic complexes. Johnson's preference rules, a way of segmenting music through chords, sonorities, and fields, parallels the material from his dissertation.

48.   ____. "Minimalism: Aesthetic, Style, or Technique?" *The Musical Quarterly* 78, no. 4 (1994): 742–73.

Johnson untangles various definitions of minimalism that appear in music historical and analytical literature. Johnson believes that minimalism can be described as an aesthetic, style, or technique; each of these terms is appropriate yet points to a specific stage in the development of minimalism. This article has been influential to Adams scholarship because it situates the composer's music within the development of the minimalist period. Early minimal pieces, whose focus aims at bringing musical processes to the surface, or pieces that lack goal-directedness, are said to exemplify a minimalist aesthetic. Music as a style, on the other hand, is a characteristic primarily in pieces from the 1970s that do not focus exclusively on creating a self-evident aural process in the manner of earlier works. Musical form during this period can incorporate different unrelated sections. To describe minimalism as a technique, Johnson states it contains musical elements used in combination (of two or more) by minimalists: repetitive rhythms, continuous form, interlocking patterns and pulses, a simple diatonic language, slow harmonic rhythm, and a lack of extended melody. Most of Adams's works fit the third category, where the composer adopts textural, harmonic, and rhythmic ideas or "techniques" while not being tied down to strict minimalist procedures. Adams's technique of extended melodies in *Harmonielehre* and other works sets him apart from the founders of minimalism.

49.   Kapusta, John. "The Self-Actualization of John Adams." *Journal of the Society for American Music* 12, no. 3 (2018): 317–44.

Musicologist Kapusta argues that John Adams embodies Abraham Maslow's notion of the self-actualized person. Kapusta chronicles the arts and culture movement in the San Francisco Bay area during the 1970s that was driven by the ideal of self-actualization. The author reveals some evidence to support his findings. First, in a concert given by Adams and the *New Music Ensemble* on April 15, 1977, the composer provided audience members with program notes that express familiar themes from Maslowian psychology. Second, the composer Charlemagne Palestine, who appropriated Maslow's notions of ecstasy and the carnal body to the music realm, gave a San Francisco performance in 1977 with *New Music Ensemble* at the invitation of Adams. Maslow argued that composers who tap into their higher unconscious could achieve peak experiences that confirm one's sense of individuality.

Kapusta seeks to demonstrate how Maslowian ideals shaped Adams's postminimalist idiom. He contributes to the definition of postminimalism as it applies to Adams, stating that it entails not only eclecticism but also a desire to "make music a medium of peak experience and self-actualization" (318). Kapusta illustrates excerpts from *Shaker Loops* as a case study, drawing parallels to Reich's modules and asserting that the loosening of compositional structures (as also noted by K. Robert Schwarz) resembles Palestine's works more closely, thereby implying full allegiance to Maslow. The author attempts to demonstrate how Adams steers away from the Reichian model by subverting meter and using unpredictable rhythmic patterns. Rather, Adams's *Shaker Loops* evokes peak experiences, as referenced in its punning title. Lastly, Kapusta explores works subsequent to *Shaker Loops*, such as *Harmonium*, and subjects them through the lens of Maslow. Kapusta interprets Adams's counsel on composition, "throwing away the compass," to mean embracing erotic and physical energy (334). Overall, the author presents a novel look at Adams's aesthetic development. Yet an equally plausible account comes directly from Adams, who proclaims his musical aesthetic combines post-Romantic ideals with minimalist techniques. On the subject of psychology, Adams himself has acknowledged influence from Jungian principles, which would seem to be at odds with Maslow's concept of growth through self-actualization. Thus, future inquiry could explore Adams's influence from Jungian psychology.

50.   Karolyi, Otto. "The Minimalists: La Monte Young, Terry Riley, Steve Reich, Philip Glass and John Adams." In *Modern American Music: From Charles Ives to the Minimalists*, 101–19. London: Cygnus Arts, 1996.

The late Karolyi traces the origins of minimalist music to minimalist art and popular music. Karolyi draws comparisons between jazz and the development of minimalism during the 1960s and early 70s. These two musical styles were motivated by the prospect of anti-establishment and disseminated in unconventional ways: jazz was performed in bars, nightclubs, and other venues, and minimalism was popularized through private performances in galleries and exhibitions. Karolyi asserts that Adams is only partially a minimalist because he prefers to intertwine romantic elements in his works. Karolyi believes that composers like Adams and Glass trigger a primordial response that is unparalleled in modernist musical movements. Following a short biography of the composer, Karolyi provides a synopsis of various musical works from Adams's oeuvre. According to Karolyi, Adams's gate works begin to reveal Adams's compositional style, showing a penchant for modality, pulsation, and subtle rhythmic and melodic patterns, but unlike other minimalists, Adams's works feature through-composed formal types. In addition to providing a synopsis of Adams's larger works, such as *Nixon in China*, Karolyi contends that this opera is more than a "caricature of the rapprochement between American and China" because it explores an aspect of human tragedy (117). On the subject of *The Death of Klinghoffer*, Karolyi does not discuss its contentious nature directly, though he takes a stance by hailing Adams as a compassionate witness.

51.   Keller, Johanna. "Resurrection Symphony." *Symphony* (League of American Orchestras) 54 (March–April 2003): 44–8.

This author contends that Adams and other contemporary composers are invoking religious contexts in their larger orchestral works. Keller discusses Adams's *El Niño*. The author notes that Adams's multilingual version of the Christmas story serves as a metaphor for a faith that crosses boundaries of culture and class. Keller briefly compares Adams's nativity oratorio to Osvaldo Golijov's telling of Christ in *La Pasión según San Marcos*. The article is supplemented with a discography of the contemporary works introduced by Keller.

52.   Kleppinger, Stanley V. "Metrical Issues in John Adams's *Short Ride in a Fast Machine*." *Indiana Theory Review* 22, no. 1 (2001): 65–81.

Kleppinger underscores the rhythmic and metrical complexity of Adams's *Short Ride in a Fast Machine*. The author provides two plausible interpretations for perceiving metrical issues in this work by grouping listeners into two groups, conservative and radical. According to Kleppinger, conservative listeners are more inclined to hear Adams's notated simple triple meter that is established from the onset by the opening woodblocks amidst conflicting textures in the clarinets and trumpets. In the more radical interpretation, listeners' perception of the meter is altered due to the increased activity in the opening trumpet part. Kleppinger devises a metrical narrative that travels through a number of perceived meters during the opening of the work. The author's narrative coincides with Adams's source of inspiration for the work, which deals with the experience of riding on a family member's new Ferrari.

53. Koay, Kheng Keow. "Baroque Minimalism in John Adams's Violin Concerto." *Tempo* 66, no. 260 (2012): 23–33.

Koay investigates the influence of Baroque music on minimalist techniques in Adams's Violin Concerto. Koay defends his study by resorting to Adams's own words on the second and third movements as being tropes from the past; namely, a *Chaconne* and *Toccata*. Koay relates the notion of musical repetition to both repertoires and illustrates how Baroque pieces can be highly repetitive. Adams, too, has acknowledged similarities in their motoric rhythm and periodic nature. According to Koay, Adams emulates a variety of Baroque musical idioms: musical sequences, common to Vivaldi and others; walking bass lines, stylistically reminiscent of Corelli and his contemporaries; a soloist cadenza with idiomatic violin techniques; the use of the "Lombard Snap," a standard Baroque short-long rhythmic pattern; and the performance practice of *notes inégales*, characteristic of French Baroque rhythmic gestures. Koay demonstrates how Adams's Violin Concerto is comprised of several musical styles, including rhythmic figures suggestive of jazz in the third movement. Koay concludes by elaborating on jazz and popular vernacular styles and influences that are inherent to the concerto and help define Adams's eclectic approach to composition.

54. Kraft, Leo. "The Death of Klinghoffer." *Perspectives of New Music* 30, no. 1 (1992): 300–2.

Kraft, an American composer and educator, writes a brief commentary on Adams's opera *The Death of Klinghoffer*. The author opines the collaboration between Peter Sellars, Alice Goodman, and John Adams results in a remarkably successful opera, one that hails a new genre of writing that will have a lasting effect. Kraft praises Adams's artistry for inventing ways of prolonging harmonies to enable the underpinning for grand musical gestures essential for a dramatic work. On a negative note, Kraft remarks that the opera shows insensitivity to Jewish audiences by portraying the American Jewish characters in a condescending manner. Kraft's condemnation of the opera's characterization of the Jewish characters has been echoed by musicologist Richard Taruskin since his 2001 *New York Times* article "Music's Dangers and the Case for Control."

55. Kramer, Lawrence. "The Great American Opera: *Klinghoffer, Streetcar*, and the Exception." *The Opera Quarterly* 23, no. 1 (2007): 66–80.

Kramer examines how music narrative and artistic aims conjoin with questions of national character in Adams's *The Death of Klinghoffer* and another recent opera by André Previn titled *A Streetcar Named Desire*. Kramer indicates that these two operas are strikingly different on the surface, yet their dramatic mode identically seeks to become "a fragment of a cycle of myths about America's character and destiny" by including the same kinds of archetypes that evoke national imagery (70). Kramer remarks that Adams's *Klinghoffer* pairs with *Nixon in China* and *Doctor Atomic* in giving a reflection of national mythology. This sense of national identity is formed through its American characters, such as the Klinghoffers, and through a charge of nostalgia. The author reflects on the *Klinghoffer* controversy, though his conclusions are markedly different from Taruskin or Fink, who stand at opposite ends of the spectrum (see items 38 and 246). Kramer is sympathetic to both sides of the argument, and he posits that one of the scenes at the forefront of the controversy, regarded as the "Rumors scene," intertwines elements of traditional Jewish humor with anti-Semitic satire, thereby blurring distinctions. Furthering the exploration of *Klinghoffer* and the controversies that surround the opera, Kramer addresses Woolcock's 2003 film production, offering a scathing critique of the film's added narratives and numerous other changes. The author draws comparisons between Leon Klinghoffer and Porgy from Gershwin's iconic American opera, situating Adams in a historical continuum of opera tradition.

56.   _____. "Like Falling Leaves: The Erotics of Mourning in Four *Drum-Taps* Settings." In *Walt Whitman and Modern Music: War, Desire, and the Trials of Nationhood*, 151–65. New York: Garland Publishing, 2000.

The author explores several musical settings of Walt Whitman's *Drum-Taps* (1865), a cycle of American Civil War poems, including John Adams's *The Wound-Dresser* for baritone, as well as others by Vaughan Williams, Rorem, and Kramer himself. Kramer expresses Whitman's views on war along with Adams's interpretation of the poems using his musical setting as a focal point. Kramer remarks that unlike most of Whitman's *Drum-Taps*, his poem "The Wound Dresser" does not touch on a single moment of mortal intimacy; rather, it gives a recollection of death in old age. According to Kramer, Adams delineates these recollections of war and death by breaking up the text in distinct formal sections, with each characterized by a distinguishable orchestral texture. Kramer remarks that Adams's setting enhances Whitman's poem and portrays the act of caring for wounded soldiers as one of consolation and commemoration. He offers a persuasive interpretation of textural relations, probing into Adams's use of repetition used at the midpoint of the song. Kramer also explores Adams's instrumentation and views the interaction between the violin and trumpet as transcendental and mysterious, imbuing them with specific affective qualities that are contrasted with the baritone solo as a reminder of the soldier's corporeal existence.

57.   Kreutziger-Herr, Annette. "Politik und Postmoderne: Die Oper *Nixon in China* von John Adams." *Hamburger Jahrbuch für Musikwissenschaft* 17 (2000): 323–50. In German.

Kreutziger-Herr explores metanarratives and political myths in *Nixon in China*. The author purports that John Cage's *Europeras* (1987) set the stage for contemporary operas likes *Nixon*. Kreutziger-Herr incorporates musical excerpts from the opening act, reminiscent to Wagner's *Rheingold*, and several other passages. She considers the state of contemporary American opera and politics with a focus on China-United States relations. Moreover, Kreutziger-Herr contrasts contemporary operas from the United States with those composed in Germany, where world premieres are funded by the government. She elaborates on Adams's biographical data and formative musical influences, and she introduces several of Adams's earlier works. The author accompanies her study with various interviews featuring Adams, previously published in English by other writers.

58.   Kühnel, Jürgen. " 'Erfolgsteams' des zeitgenössischen Musiktheaters: Robert Wilson und Philip Glass/Philip Glass und Achim Freyer/John Adams und Peter Sellars; 'Multimedia-Oper' und 'CNN opera.'" In *Musiktheater der Gegenwart: Text und Komposition, Rezeption und Klangbildung*, eds. Jürgen Kühnel, Ulrich Müller, and Oswald Panagl, 536–54. Anif: Verlag Mueller-Speiser, 2008.

Kühnel discusses the collaboration between Adams and Sellars in *Nixon in China*, *The Death of Klinghoffer*, *I Was Looking at the Ceiling and Then I Saw the Sky*, *El Niño*, and *Doctor Atomic*. Kühnel posits that Glass's *Einstein on the Beach* paved the way for a genre of media opera continued by Adams's *Nixon*, and outside the United States, by Gerhard Rosenfeld's *Kniefall in Warsaw*. To this aim, Kühnel provides comparisons between Glass and Adams. The author also points to American theater, especially Broadway musicals, as a precedent for minimalist opera. Kühnel provides a brief summary of Adams's second opera and discusses its troubled reception among music critics and scholars. The author does the same for Adams's 1995 "song play," noting Adams and Sellars's dramaturgy is reminiscent of Robert Altman's 1993 film *Short Cuts*, without going into detail. Kühnel offers interesting references to other operas and films as they relate to the Adams-Sellars collaboration, though the article primarily serves to introduce German readers to Adams's stage works.

59.   Laki, Peter. "Two Operatic Oppenheimer's." *Ars Lyrica: Journal of the Lyrica Society for Word-Music Relations* 25 (forthcoming).

Laki compares Adams's depiction of Oppenheimer in *Doctor Atomic* to that of composer István Anhalt, who began writing an opera on Oppenheimer for the Canadian Opera Company over a decade before Adams (for a preliminary comparison of these two operas, see item 19). For various reasons outlined in Laki's study, Anhalt's project never came to fruition. Nevertheless, many of the files and sketches preserved at Library Archives Canada were sealed until 2012. The two operas have eight characters in total, though Anhalt includes the psychiatrist and physician Jean Tatlock. One of the most poignant moments of Adams's opera is when Oppenheimer sings an aria composed from John Donne's sonnet "Batter my heart, three-person'd God." Laki explains that Anhalt also set Donne's poem in his libretto, though at the conclusion of a scene between Oppenheimer and Tatlock, a scene that contains premonitions of the future. Laki compares the portrayal of other shared characters, including Kitty Oppenheimer, Edward Teller, and General Groves. Laki concludes by stating that the ultimate aim of each composer was invariably different: Anhalt employed historical analogies from the past using Jewish overtones, while Adams and Sellars gave Oppenheimer a mythical dimension.

60.   Lee, Christopher. "Rhythm and the Cold War Imaginary: Listening to John Adams's *Nixon in China.*" *Differences: A Journal of Feminist Cultural Studies* 22, no. 2–3 (2011): 190–210.

Lee introduces theories from postmodernism to explain the conflict between capitalism and communism. He offers an analysis of *Nixon in China* as an artifact of the Cold War, namely, to show how Adams's use of rhythm reveals the limits of global imagery on the verge of disintegration. Lee's larger aim is to elucidate how Adams's *Nixon in China* engages with the limits of its own ideological parameters. The author posits that Adams's opera registers the anxieties between American and Chinese ideologies by tracing Nixon's journey through a minimalist musical idiom. Moreover, Lee aims to show how *Nixon's* minimalist aesthetic, particularly in regards to its temporal aspects, merges with the subject matter and narrative. The first encounter between Nixon and Mao in the opera contains rhythmically juxtaposed vocal lines between the two leaders, which convey their difficulty in communicating. The music slows considerably as Premier Chou En-lai brings up Mao's doctrines as commentary that class conflict is unavoidable in socialist ideology. The librettist Goodman rewords these claims into a meditation on revolution and time, and Adams halts the pulse-driven music on the word "duration." Lee examines other moments of the opera where the libretto, the music, and the sense of time appear to be at the foreground. In his conclusion, Lee asserts that the opera's use of sound and rhythm generates ambivalence and "undermine[s] expectations of formal or narrative closure stemming from the opera's ideological and thematic materials" (206).

61.   Longobardi, Ruth Sara. "Re-producing *Klinghoffer*: Opera and Arab Identity Before and After 9/11." *Journal of the Society for American Music* 3, no. 3 (2009): 273–310.

Longobardi traces initial reviews of Adams's *The Death of Klinghoffer* premiere, whose common thread voiced the work's failure to portray the hijackers as terrorists and instead regard them as victims of Israeli aggression. Longobardi researches media and source material on the *Achille Lauro* hijacking, including two television movies preceding the opera itself, a memoir written by the ship's captain, a variety of published analytical texts, and broadcast and print news media. Longobardi applies Bill Nichols's film theory of three axes of representation, which informs the narrative plot development, historical references, and myths and spectacles.

Longobardi proposes that pre- and post-9/11 productions of *Klinghoffer* represented the Palestinian hijackers in a divergent manner. In earlier productions of the opera, its creators paint the subject of terrorism with ambiguity, inviting dialogue on the Israeli-Palestinian conflict. Conversely, post-9/11 productions rely on film and photographs, thereby highlighting racial differences and denouncing its perpetrators. One post-9/11 example entails Bob McGrath's production, which presents the tragic events in a more factual fashion and gives closure to the opera as a way to accommodate for more sensitive audiences affected by the devastation of September 11. The remainder of Longobardi's study explores revisions and reconstructions of the opera and presents musical examples for further analysis of the ramifications of the collaborators' revisions.

62. Margulis, Elizabeth Hellmuth. "An Exploratory Study of Narrative Experiences of Music." *Music Perception* 35, no. 2 (2017): 235–48.

Margulis develops an empirical music-cognition study that explores the likelihood listeners might concoct a subjective narrative while listening to instrumental music ranging from the Baroque era to the minimalist style. Margulis defends her study as one among a host of writings—including music philosopher Peter Kivy and theorist Byron Almén—that explore narrativity in instrumental music. The author selects musical excerpts exhibiting a high degree of contrast from nineteenth- and early twentieth-century repertoire, while excerpts with low contrast were chosen from Baroque and minimalist repertoire. The representative minimalist works include Terry Riley's *In C* and John Adams's *Shaker Loops*. Participants in the study were asked a variety of questions to gauge their engagement with the music. Margulis's questionnaire, included in an appendix, is geared to measure narrative understanding, attentional focus, narrative presence, and emotional engagement. Additionally, brief personality tests were conducted to categorize participants into introverted or extraverted personality types. Margulis concludes that Adams's *Shaker Loops* elicits a higher number of participant narratives than Riley's *In C*, though not to the extent of Romantic repertoire. In the majority of responses about *Shaker Loops*, participants described its emotive qualities with action words such as *racing, running, riding*, or *dashing*. Diverging from the Baroque repertoire in the study, which gave participants a temporal orientation of the past, Adams's minimalist work elicits a narrative associated with the future. Margulis's approach to music cognition reveals noteworthy findings of Adams's early *Shaker Loops*, yet the broad corpus under study and its small sampling of minimalist works leaves room for future inquiry on minimalist composers.

63. Masnikosa, Marija. "A Theoretical Model of Postminimalism and Two Brief 'Case Studies.'" In *The Ashgate Research Companion to Minimalist and Postminimalist Music*, eds. Keith Potter, Kyle Gann, and Pwyll Ap Siôn, 297–311. Farnham: Ashgate Publishing Limited, 2013.

Masnikosa devotes the first portion of her book chapter to define the principal characteristics of minimalism and postminimalism. Her understanding of the minimalist style is supported by other writers' notions of the development of the compositional style: namely, Kyle Gann and Paul Epstein. The difference for

Gann lies on whether listeners can perceive an audible structure. Epstein believes that when a composer's will is perceptible, that conscious choice of writing lies within the postminimalist style. Masnikosa characterizes minimalist music as a highly rigid process of composition that lacks strong contrast, maintains a certain absence of musical expression, features slow-moving harmonic progressions, and shuns a hierarchy of repetitions and minimalist textures. Masnikosa's theoretical model for minimalist works includes various stages. The first entails analysis of the work in regards to its compositional process and an examination of its repetitive structures. The second stage derives a close reading of a musical work through semiotics. This aids in recognizing non-minimalist segments integrated within postminimalist works. The third stage aims to identify and interpret referential signs in the work.

The second case study of the author's theoretical model presents Adams's *Harmonielehre*. Masnikosa considers the work postminimalist, partly due to the second movement's tripartite form and less repetitive nature. Some of the defining characteristics of the work include "explicit modular repetition, phase shifting or, in some passages, permutational (and isorhythmic) repetition of small sets of pitch classes" (307). Masnikosa clarifies an interesting aspect of Adams's work. While the work as a whole contains semantically coded postminimalist textures, they are contrasted with non-hierarchically arranged minimalist textures. Yet another contrasting factor between minimalist and postminimalist features pertains to the vertical structures, which include simultaneous sounding layers and drones. In minimalist passages, the vertical structures unfold calmly with minimal contrast, while in postminimalist sections harmonic development offers greater contrast. Masnikosa includes several musical excerpts, highlighting the manner in which harmonic textures blend with melodic lines. Continuing the discussion of the middle movement, Masnikosa asserts that the presentation of harmonic collection differs from the outer movements as it keeps changing while not maintaining a certain number of pitches in common. The author claims that in some sections of the movement the melodic lines are derived mostly from the existing harmonic structure, while in contrapuntal portions of the movement, Adams's melodic lines are mostly independent of the aggregate vertical structures. According to Masnikosa, these independent notes have a floating quality that discursively stands apart from the repetitive discourse surrounding them.

In the next stage of her analysis, Masnikosa examines referential aspects of *Harmonielehre*, such as the reference to Schoenberg in the title and subtitles for the second and third movements. Adams's melodies allude to Wagner, though specific quotations are not apparent. Masnikosa asserts that at the semantic level, Adams's style finds its home in *fin de siècle* European tradition, with its Mahlerian sighs, Schoenbergian long climaxes, and Wagnerian tendency to prolong harmonic tension. In her conclusion, Masnikosa reiterates her earlier point that the origins of the postminimalist style are brought on by the composer's voice and the presence of agency.

64.   May, Thomas. "*A Flowering Tree*: The Composer, The Music." *Jung Journal: Culture and Psyche* 2 (2008): 41–8.

May provides background information of Adams's opera *A Flowering Tree*, including its date of composition, commission (to commemorate the 250th anniversary of Mozart's birth), synopsis (adapted from an ancient tale of Indian origin), world premiere, performers, collaboration with Sellars, and an interest in writing multilingual dramatic works. May is convinced that Adams's recent works are neither minimalist nor neo-Romantic. Adams's efforts to capture the spirit of Mozart continue to propel his works with a yin and yang impetus from the serious (*Doctor Atomic*) to the lighthearted (*A Flowering Tree*). Adams's style of melodic writing with frequent wide intervals pays homage to *El Niño*. May examines text-music relations from the narrator and two principal characters. May contrasts Kumudha's tree transformations with Richard Strauss's transformation music in *Daphne*: the former occurs throughout the opera, rather than at the final climax. The author observes that Adams sets Kumudha's transformations to static A-minor harmonies—another salutary reference to Adams's early opera, *Nixon*. May gives much importance to Adams's *Flores* chorus because it assumes a more important role than the typical Greek chorus commenting on the action. This topic has been explored in Linell Gray Moss's 1998 work "The Chorus as Character in Three American Operas of the Late Twentieth Century," who addresses many of the same points in Adams's *The Death of Klinghoffer* (see item 170).

65.   ____. "John Adams' Development as a Composer Can Be Charted in String Music." *Strings Magazine* 272 (December 2017): 22–5.

May asserts that string music has played a defining role in Adams's compositional development. The author looks to *Shaker Loops* as the primary springboard for Adams's preoccupation for string writing. He cites prominent string works Adams has composed since *John's Book of Alleged Dances*, including his String Quartet No. 1 from 2008 and String Quartet No. 2 from 2014. May draws parallels to Camille Saint-Saëns for embarking on compositions for strings later in life. Listening to the St. Lawrence String Quartet play a Beethoven string quartet piqued Adams's interest to compose string works and even include musical references to Beethoven. May echoes Adams's stance on his stylistic influences; namely, minimalism is simply one technique in his toolbox. May's assertion that Adams's Violin Concerto was his antidote for exploring outside of minimalism toward a more melodic style is off the mark. The minimalist underpinning of *Nixon in China* forced Adams to elevate the parameter of melody as an equal partner in the music-making process, resulting in a variety of new kinds of works, such as *Eros Piano*, *The Death of Klinghoffer*, and the Chamber Symphony. Nevertheless, May's topic is evidenced by the fact that Adams has concentrated on writing for strings to a greater degree than other solo instruments.

66.   Miller, Malcolm. "From Liszt to Adams: The 'Wiegenlied' Transcription." *Tempo* New Series 175 (1990): 23–6.

Miller examines Adams's arrangement for chamber orchestra of Liszt's *Wie-genlied* for piano, which originated from his last tone poem, *Von der Weige bis zum Grabe*. Miller posits that numerous similarities between Liszt's work and the minimalist style may have prompted Adams to create his own arrangement, including using fragmentary motivic content, harmonic ambiguity, and the repetition of rhythms and intervals. According to Miller, Adams's use of timbre serves three functions: (1) coloristic, to project its atmosphere; (2) structural, to highlight aspects of form; and (3) stylistic, to imbue the music with a minimalist style. It is probable that this transcription and others from this period served Adams as a basis for experimentation in writing instrumental music and seeking a new compositional voice that resulted in his large orchestral works.

67.   _____. "From Liszt to Adams (II): 'The Black Gondola." *Tempo* New Series 179 (1991): 17–20.

Miller discusses John Adams's chamber orchestra transcription of Liszt's late piano work *La Lugubre Gondola II*. Liszt claimed to have a premonition of Wagner's death in Venice, and thus the motivic content of the work includes the opening them of *Tristan und Isolde*. Miller asserts that Adams's orchestration operates at structural, stylistic, and poetic levels. Before approaching the reprise or return of the opening thematic section, Adams reinterprets the original musical textures with arpeggio figures akin to a minimalist style. The poetic element is inherent in Adams's programmatic approach to The Black Gondola, using special effects like harmonics, mutes, and tuning string instruments down a semitone.

68.   Noubel, Max. "L'ère du post-stylisme selon John Adams: Savant populaire ou populisme savant?" In *Musique savante et musique populaire aux États-Unis: XXe et XXIe siècles*, 91–104. Dijon: Editions Universitaires de Dijon, 2017. In French.

An English translation of Noubel's article reads as "The Post-Style Era According to John Adams: Popular Classicist or Classical Populism?" Noubel asserts that Adams's flirtations with popular music blur the lines between noble and trivial, scholarly and popular. Noubel references an interview where Adams describes himself as a post-style composer. The author explores the classical and popular synthesis in Adams's works in light of minimalism, Duke Ellington, Romanticism in *Nixon in China*, the influence of Copland's *Rodeo* in *Gnarly Buttons*, and *Fanfare for the Common Man* in *Short Ride in a Fast Machine*. Adams's blend between classical tradition and popular culture also influences his approach to writing melody. The simplicity of melodic lines in *John's Book of Alleged Dances* resembles popular music, whereas modulations and sophisticated turns of phrases point towards the classical tradition. Noubel touches upon other popular elements of Adams's music, including instrumentation, extroverted qualities, and the impression of wide-open spaces emblematic of the American landscape.

69.   Novak, Jelena. "From Minimalist Music to Postopera: Repetition, Representation and (Post)Modernity in the Operas of Philip Glass and Louis Andriessen." In *The Ashgate Research Companion to Minimalist and Postminimalist Music*, eds.

Keith Potter, Kyle Gann, and Pwyll Ap Siôn, 129–40. Farnham: Ashgate Publishing Limited, 2013.

Novak writes on the integration of the minimalist style in opera music, focusing predominantly on Glass and Andriessen. Her study also gives a relevant picture of the stylistic development that led to operatic writing in these two composers and also Reich and Adams. Novak posits that minimalism's foray into the opera world coincided with its abandonment of modernism. The shift from minimalism correlates with three significant historical changes: transitioning from minimalist to postminimalist music, from opera to *postopera*, and from modernism to postmodernism. This more mature form of minimalism moved the non-narrative mechanisms used in repetitive music to narrative genres. Novak defines postminimalism as a heterogeneous conceptual field where composers reinterpret and question minimalism in their music. The author also concurs with Timothy Johnson's own view of minimalism as a technique. Postopera has bloomed as a result of the digitization of opera performances and the confluence of film, visual arts, video, and theater. Novak's term *postopera* applies to John Adams's operas because they are contemporary, non-conventional, and postmodern. In these works, the relationship between music and drama is reinvented and impacted by new media.

70.   _____. "Televisual Opera After TV." In *Das Wohnzimmer als Loge. Von der Fernsehoper zum medialen Musiktheater*, eds. Matthias Henke and Sara Beimdieke, 179–96. Würzburg: Königshausen & Neumann, 2016.

This book contains chapters in German and English, the latter of which include Novak's examination of operas succeeding the age of television, including Adams and Sellars's "CNN operas." The author remarks how new media in opera has diversified its spectatorship. Novak asserts that this new television opera genre has affected the way contemporary operas are structured. Furthermore, the unfolding drama of Adams's operas questions the medium of news in a televised format. While Novak concurs that Adams and Sellars's works explore aspects of the events not televised, she also opines that Sellars's staging decisions are largely dominated by television and newspaper sources. More recent productions, however, depart from Sellars's initial objectives.

71.   Ortiz, Mario A. "Sor Juana en *El Niño* de John Adams y *Óyeme con los ojos* de Allison Sniffin." *Cuadernos de música, artes visuales y artes escénicas* 4, no. 1–2 (2008): 207–34. In Spanish.

Ortiz explores the musical representation of Sor Juana in *El Niño* and a cantata by Allison Sniffin. Adams set two religious texts by Sor Juana in *El Niño* (the *villancicos* titled "Pues mi Dios a nacido a penar" and "Por celebrar del Infante"), keeping the original text in Spanish. The author elucidates how Adams's depiction differs radically from the protofeminist and subversive portrayal more commonly found in recent decades. According to Ortiz, Adams celebrates Sor Juana's religious views as an author of Christmas carols. Ortiz contrasts the visual artwork included in the CD cover—Yreina D. Cervantes's serigraph of Sor Juana titled *Mujer de mucha enagua*—to Adams's own musical depiction. The author asserts that Cervantes's artwork presents a feminist and political discourse that departs from Adams's own musical treatment. Ortiz gives a detailed interpretation of the painting and explains that Cervantes's Sor Juana is subversive because she transcends time, sharing visual space with two other historical figures from different epochs. Cervantes's Sor Juana speaks in Nahuatl, Mexico's principal indigenous language. In contrast, Adams's Sor Juana speaks Castilian exclusively, adheres to poetic conventions of Spanish Christmas carols, and does not portray her protofeminist, Latin-American positions. According to Ortiz, the inclusion of Cervantes's artwork is not coincidental; Sellars affirms that it influenced the conception of *El Niño*.

72.   Pellegrino, Catherine. "Aspects of Closure in the Music of John Adams." *Perspectives of New Music* 40, no. 1 (2002): 147–75.

Pellegrino explores aspects of closure in Adams's *Phrygian Gates* and *The Chairman Dances*. The author considers three categories for establishing closure: tonal organization, formal aspects, and rhetorical elements. Closure in Adams's works takes on a different form than the traditional tonal models, whereby harmonies gravitate towards a reference point. Pellegrino asserts that postmodern methodologies of musical analysis are better suited to open a window into the composer's techniques than traditional, formalist analysis. In *Phrygian Gates*, tonal organization is perceived by the gradual mutation of harmonic structures through a repeated cyclical process until the music reverts to its point of origin. Formal aspects of closure are reliant on other types of closure. Rhetorical elements, like an intensification (or reduction) of orchestral textures, dynamics, and register, are an effective method of closure in Adams's compositions. Pellegrino also offers commentary on the nature of postmodernism and the aspects of Adams's music that fit the aesthetic.

73.   Powell, Richard. "Accessible Narratives: Continuity in the Music of John Adams." *Contemporary Music Review* 33, no. 4 (2014): 390–407.

Powell explores the notion of continuity in John Adams's works using *Shaker Loops* and *Harmonielehre* as case studies. The author asserts that Adams's postminimalist style draws the audience to the act of listening in its most fundamental way. Musical continuity is investigated from various perspectives, using notions such as diversity, motion, space, gravity, convergence, divergence, and crystallization. According to Powell, *Harmonielehre* achieves a synthesis of styles, including post-Romantic, impressionist, and Schoenbergian influences, infused under the umbrella of minimalism. Powell posits that such a diverse narrative leads to a heightened sense of continuity. In place of tightly woven compositional design, Adams creates shifting narratives, aided by tempo, dynamics, and the underlying textures. In *Shaker Loops*, the modular sequences serve as leitmotifs, and their transformations contribute to their continuity. Powell states that musical continuity in *Harmonielehre* can be observed by studying the kinds of musical gestures evident in the work, and to this aim, the author creates various graphs to track the entire work, including a gestural graph that shows points of intensity and a tempo graph that charts the changing of gears throughout the work. In regards to musical space, Powell considers Adams's dream images of the work and how they are reflected as space and motion. The author equates the notion of gravity to tonal centeredness. According to Powell, while *Shaker Loops* is conceived using diatonic constructs, one could argue that its first movement is driven by a series of tonal centers that emerge, overlap, conflict, or fade, resulting in a dialogue between gravitational fields.

74. Ramaut-Chevassus, Béatrice. "Arnold Schoenberg, une reference pour John Adams." *Ostinato Rigore* 17, no. 1 (2001): 293–307. In French.

Ramaut-Chevassus explores stylistic convergences between Schoenberg and Adams in light of their profoundly different aesthetics. The author describes a link between the two composers following the lineage from Schoenberg's pupil, Leon Kirchner, who later became Adams's teacher at Harvard. According to this author, Adams's *Harmonielehre* and his Chamber Symphony represent outward references to Schoenberg. The author posits the goal of these two works is to achieve a synthesis between twentieth-century theory and practice and to evoke the language of Schoenberg. Ramaut-Chevassus believes both composers are fascinated with nostalgia. In the case of Adams, he seeks to inject pure minimalism with emotion. Schoenberg believed that every composer aspires to return to an older style. Ramaut-Chevassus devotes her concluding portion to the importance of visual imagery for Schoenberg and Adams. The former regards composition as the art of simple imitation of nature. Inspiration for Adams is nourished by dream images that he consciously molds into a new work.

75. ____. "La pratique citationnelle, puissance ou impuissance pour l'œuvre musicale? L'exemple de John Adams." In *Fragment, montage-démontage, collage-décollage, la défection de l'œuvre?* eds. Jean-Paul Olive and Claude Amey, 119–30. Paris: L'Harmattan, 2004. In French.

Ramaut-Chevassus explores the practice of musical quotation as a signature trait of the postmodern era. The author considers Adams's thoughts on popular music, offers specific references to Adams's musical quotations, and describes their function within the minimalist aesthetic. Ramaut-Chevassus gives a succinct overview of quotation in Adams's oeuvre, focusing on many of the composer's top hits, including Chamber Symphony and the more recent works *El Niño* and *On the Transmigration of Souls*.

76. Reilly, Robert R. "John Adams: The Search for a Larger Harmony." In *Surprised by Beauty: A Listener's Guide to the Recovery of Modern Music*, 29–35. San Francisco: Ignatius, 2016.

In the opening chapter from this listener's guide to modern music, Reilly explores Adams's compositional style and musical works. Its intended readership is geared toward those unfamiliar with Adams's works. Concerning the earlier works such as *Harmonium*, Reilly commends Adams's separation from atonality despite having been indoctrinated in the dodecaphonic system of composition during his Harvard days. Reilly cites portions from an interview with Adams, surmising that *El Niño* is a contemporary affirmation of faith. Reilly notes the title of Adams's oratorio underwent bouts of uncertainty. It was initially entitled *How Could This Happen?*, subsequently *Nativité* for its Paris premiere, and in the end, its collaborators settled on *El Niño*. Reilly criticizes Adams and Sellars's choice of text from the Gnostic Gospels, claiming the collaborators took many liberties in their depictions rather than setting a more traditional account of the nativity. Reilly opines that Adams fails to answer the question posed by the original title *How could this happen?* and believes the more pertinent questions should be "what happened, and who is Christ"? For the remainder of the chapter, Reilly reviews Adams's post-*Nixon in China* works, including *On the Transmigration of Souls* and *My Father Knew Charles Ives*.

77.   Renihan, Colleen. "Gesture, Temporality, and the Politics of Engagement in Opera Film." *Music, Sound, and the Moving Image* 8, no. 1 (2014): 57–85.

Renihan explores Penny Woolcock's 2003 film rendering of Adams's *The Death of Klinghoffer*. The author examines Woolcock's film images vis-à-vis Adams's minimalist score, touching upon the work's manipulation of traditional notions of subjectivity in opera. The author asserts that the film provides the viewer with opportunities for further engagement with political themes central to Adams's opera. Renihan's article looks back to Woolcock's first exposure to excerpts from Adams's opera performed at the Barbican and considers her collaboration with Adams's *Doctor Atomic* as director of the production performed by the Metropolitan Opera. Woolcock's opinion of Adams's *Klinghoffer* reveals her reconciliatory efforts between the conflicting sides. Renihan treats some key topics independently: positioning the viewer, the "Aria of the Falling Body," and narrative disjuncture and cultural resonances. The author explores ways in which Woolcock's film is a stark contrast to the original stage production of *Klinghoffer*, which downplays distinctions between Israeli and Palestinian characters. The author studies portions of Adams's score that examine the crucial ending scene in the opera and offers a comparison with Bach's aria "Erbarme Dich" from the *St Matthew Passion*. Renihan elaborates on Bach's aria and elucidates parallels between Bach and Adams's arias, most notably, the way in which subjective identification from Bach's aria functions in Adams's *Klinghoffer*. The author's study cites some of the more significant writings on *Klinghoffer*, including Taruskin's harsh criticism of the opera and Fink's cultural studies. Furthermore, Renihan integrates concepts from music semiotics by Cumming, Hatten, and Monelle, to explore the *pianto* musical motives in Adams's aria as a way of approximating an effect similar to Bach's *obbligato* lines.

78.   Robinson, Paul. "Repetition Tropes and Levels of Obliteration in John Adams's Saxophone Concerto and *American Berserk*." *Tempo* 70, no. 277 (July 2016): 47–62.

Robinson explores two recent works by Adams that have received little analytical attention: the Saxophone Concerto and *American Berserk*. Robinson asserts that although Adams has strived to distance himself from his early minimalist tendencies (and the composer has at times even refuted being a minimalist composer), traces of minimalist techniques persist in his recent works. Namely, Adams continues to employ cyclical patterns (in the first Violin Concerto), modal and tonal materials (the Saxophone Concerto and *American Berserk*), and single patterns that extend for large spans of music (*Naive and Sentimental Music*). The slow evolution of Adams's music is an aesthetic of delayed gratification, where subtle changes can make a big impact. Robinson purports that *American Berserk* is constructed with a precompositional design, and in order to prove his point, the author employs the concept of "tropes of repetition" from Rebecca Leydon's work on minimalist tropes. Robinson identifies various themes in *American Berserk* (a four-note theme, chorale theme, and scherzo motives) and tracks their development throughout the work in tandem with his analysis of repetitive tropes.

Aside from Adams's more mature style of writing that features greater surface contrast, rhythmic and melodic variety, and tonal diversity, the Saxophone Concerto stems from a singular structural idea, which entails the transformation of the modal chords from the onset in a manner that parallels the opening of the first Violin Concerto. Robinson reproduces a short musical incipit from the Saxophone Concerto to illustrate how melodic treatment is subjected to a unifying mode of thought. According to the author, Adams's technique for melodic development is influenced by Slonimsky's *Thesaurus of Scales and Melodic Patterns*. Considering the overall structure from the first movement of the Saxophone Concerto, Robinson charts some notable formal markers, focusing on harmonic structures, repetition tropes, tempo fluctuations, and the contour of melodic and rhythmic aspects of these repetitive motives.

79.   Sanchez-Behar, Alexander. "Dovetailing in John Adams's 'Chain to the Rhythm.'" *Indiana Theory Review* 31, no. 1–2 (2013): 88–114.

This article presents an analytic study of musical dovetailing, one of Adams's signature techniques from the 1990s onwards, which entails overlapping formal sections as a means of creating smooth transitions. I examine the third movement from Adams's *Naive and Sentimental Music*, titled "Chain to the Rhythm," as a model for other recent works that feature the same technique, such as *Lollapalooza*. Analysis of dovetailing opens a window into other compositional aspects inseparable from the process of joined transitions, including closure in minimalist music, as well as motivic, harmonic, proportional, and formal features of the work. Adams's "Chain to the Rhythm" brings dovetailed transitions to the fore through dual textural and block subtractive and additive processes, joined by recurring pitch collections that mark the beginning of a new formal section. One of the most noteworthy features of Adams's "Chain to the Rhythm" is that dovetailed passages establish a direct relationship to the proportions of each formal section of the work.

80.   _____. "Finding Slonimsky's *Thesaurus of Scales and Melodic Patterns* in Two
       Concerti by John Adams." *Music Theory Spectrum* 37, no. 2 (2015): 175–88.

This article explores Adams's incorporation of symmetrical musical patterns
from Nicolas Slonimsky's *Thesaurus of Scales and Melodic Patterns* in his own
musical works. Adams has acknowledged borrowing from Slonimsky's patterns
as a source of ideas for composition, though his methodology and motivation
have remained an enigma, in part due to the complex nature of the *Thesaurus*.
Most of the melodic patterns contained in this book consist of symmetrical collections of notes, such as the hexatonic, octatonic, and enneatonic (nine note)
collections. Musical analyses of Adams's Violin Concerto and *Century Rolls* illustrate his method for integrating these symmetrical patterns. Adams's concerti
initially quote one of Slonimsky's patterns in complete form (mimicking prime
and retrograde forms), thereby acknowledging the *Thesaurus* as the original
source. Subsequently, Adams applies a series of pitch modifications and reorder-
ing of these patterns. Once Adams presents and varies a pattern, he recomposes
the pattern as his own while maintaining some resemblance to Slonimsky's patterns in their length and contour. At times Adams treats Slonimsky's *Thesaurus*
like a real book of synonyms, thereby integrating other related patterns from the
book that have similar properties in music-theoretical terms, such as the same
interval cycle, or subset and superset relations. The final portion of the article
investigates the harmonization of these patterns as prescribed by Slonimsky and
realized in Adams's concerti.

81.   _____. "Symmetry in the Music of John Adams." *Tempo* 68, no. 268 (2014): 46–60.

This article takes an analytical bend to explore the notion of symmetry in
Adams's works. Close examination of Adams's works reveals his propensity
for creating symmetrical structures throughout his compositional career. His
works from the 1970s reveal preconceived formal symmetries that influence
overall structure in pieces such as *China Gates* and *Phrygian Gates*. These early
works employ a reflectional symmetry where musical structures are main-
tained or transformed across an axis of symmetry. In the 1980s his compositional style shifts away from creating overarching symmetrical structures
in favor of symmetry at the phrase level. *Grand Pianola Music* and *Fearful
Symmetries* utilize translational symmetry, where musical phrases are restated,
at times with variation, at periodic intervals. During the 1990s Adams's interest for symmetry takes on another form, that of creating smaller symmetrical
structures at the level of motivic content. Musical textures develop through
rotational symmetry, whereby triadic transpositions and rotations in the Violin Concerto and *Century Rolls* bestow the music with a sense of coherence
and forward momentum. It is during this latest period that he begins to quote
musical patterns from Slonimsky's *Thesaurus of Scales and Melodic Patterns*,
a book that contains transpositionally symmetrical patterns organized into a
musical thesaurus.

82. Schaal, Hans-Jürgen. "Die überwindung Der Langeweile: John Adams Versöhnt Minimal Music Und Expressionismus." *Neue Zeitschrift Für Musik* 161, no. 5 (2000): 34–6. In German.

   Schaal considers how Adams reconciles minimalism and expressionism into a new aesthetic. Schaal notes that Adams regards minimalism as a style of music, not a formal dogma. The author introduces Adams's early works, honing in on *Shaker Loops*. Schaal observes that *Shaker Loops* iterates endless loops that combine into vibrant minimalist textures. However, the work's seemingly minimalist textures do not provide the impetus for the work, which exhibits expressionist traits. According to Schaal, *Shaker Loops* displays interruptions, modulations, and changes in tempo and dynamics, none of which reflect the pure minimalist style of composition. Schaal hypothesizes that minimalism arose as a reaction to integral serialism, and yet the rivalry between trance-like pulsations of major triads and the fragmentary techniques of Schoenberg's expressionist style can be reconciled. Schaal opines that Adams's Chamber Symphony exhibits a blend of atonal expressionism, jazz, and minimalism. Schaal concludes by describing shared elements between Adams and Schoenberg: abruptness, expressiveness, drama, tempo changes, and virtuosity. Thus, Adams's style has developed beyond notions of early minimalism in his search for a new mode of expression.

83. Scherzinger, Martin. "Double Voices of Musical Censorship After 9/11." In *Music in the Post-9/11 World*, eds. Jonathan Ritter and J. Martin Daughtry, 91–121. New York: Routledge, 2007.

   Scherzinger examines musical censorship following the September 11 terrorist attacks. Among the range of composers and musical works in question, the author explores Boston Symphony Orchestra's cancellation of four performances from Adams's *The Death of Klinghoffer* choruses shortly after the 9/11 attack. Scherzinger revisits the arguments made from an open-minded point of view, supported by music critic Antony Tommasini, that one of art's missions is to test limits and open perspectives, versus a more conservative opinion, prompted by musicologist Richard Taruskin, stating that the Boston Symphony Orchestra exercised good judgement and self-control for withdrawing Adams's music. Questions regarding the nature and distinction between censorship and voluntary control are at the forefront of Scherzinger's essay. The author seeks a dispassionate compromise, at times striving to bolster Taruskin's points and suggesting the musicologist might show how the Boston Symphony Orchestra acted in the best interests of the public, yet also noting that Taruskin's insistence on voluntary censorship presents a problematic stance when faced with censorship backed by law. In his conclusion, Scherzinger seems content to provide an entryway into the various debates on musical censorship.

84. Schwarz, David. "Listening Subjects: Semiotics, Psychoanalysis, and the Music of John Adams and Steve Reich." *Perspectives of New Music* 31, no. 2 (1993): 24–56.

Schwarz applies recent theories of Lacanian psychoanalytic criticism for the analysis of John Adams and Steve Reich's music. Schwarz demonstrates how psychoanalytic concepts like the *acoustic mirror* and *sonorous envelope* can be utilized to explore a connection between psychic and musical structures. The sonorous envelope refers to the maternal voice a newborn infant first hears, whereas the acoustic mirror refers to a phase of development where a baby begins to imitate sounds from the mother's voice. Schwarz describes an analogy of the sonorous envelope in the opening measures of Adams's *Nixon in China* as being devoid of dialectical relationships. The acoustic mirror is characterized by moments in which a listener recognizes indirect quotations of other composers (Schwarz and Patrick McCreless have noted some resemblance between the opening measures from *Nixon* and Wagner's opening of *Das Rheingold*). To elaborate on acoustic mirroring, Schwarz illustrates additional uses of appropriation in Adams's *Fearful Symmetries* and *Grand Pianola Music*.

85.   ____. "Music as Sonorous Envelope and Acoustic Mirror." In *Listening Subjects: Music, Psychoanalysis, Culture*, 7–22. Durham: Duke University Press, 1997.

Schwarz's book chapter presents a revised version of his 1993 article "Listening Subjects: Semiotics, Psychoanalysis, and the Music of John Adams and Steve Reich" (see item 84). Schwarz's newer study overlaps with his older publication in portions of its prose, several musical examples, and topics explored. Once again, Schwarz introduces the notion of the sonorous envelope from psychoanalytic research. In psychoanalytic terms, the sonorous envelope consists of the development of a baby's senses while in the womb and shortly after birth. Musically speaking, it draws upon first musical experiences during a person's early stages that help shape one's own musical subjectivity. The author posits that minimalist music represents the sonorous envelope as a fantasy experience and fantasy space. Specifically, the manner in which Adams employs familiar rhythmic structures and pitch content, yet in new ways, yields suitable analytical inquiry as a representation of the sonorous envelope. In this revised version of the article, Schwarz once again stresses musical precedents (which he terms "pseudoquotes") in *Nixon in China* that reference earlier classical and Romantic composers.

86.   ____. "Postmodernism, the Subject and the Real in John Adams' *Nixon in China*." *Indiana Theory Review* 13, no. 2 (1992): 107–35.

Schwarz examines *Nixon in China* by integrating the study of semiotics, which ascribes meaning to both linguistic and non-linguistic sign systems. The author attempts to reconcile his attraction to the music from *Nixon in China* with his resistance to American geo-political exploits in the opera. Schwarz posits a paradox, that the creators of the opera are both complicit and resistant to the glorification of American politics. Schwarz opines that the libretto and music subvert the sense of linear narrative due to the absence of a big finale, a climax in the plot, and a joint declaration from opposing parties. The author aims at a discursive space that can be described psychoanalytically using Jacques Lacan's concept of the Real. Schwarz asserts that *Nixon in China* negates certain aspects of traditional opera design, and in doing so, strains these conventions and conjures an image of Lacan's Real, which the author describes as something that flows into our consciousness outside of normal imagery and symbolic structures. Another topic Schwarz discusses stems from Freud's notion of the uncanny. The author employs familiar procedures from the classical tradition while eschewing the standard sequence of musical ideas, thereby creating an uncanny effect through the opposition of familiar versus non-familiar elements.

87. Schwarz, K. Robert. "Minimalism/Music." In *Perceptible Processes: Minimalism and the Baroque*, ed. Claudia Swan, 1–13. New York: Eos Music, 1997.

Schwarz presents a concise overview of the minimalist style, citing Reich for his simple but elegant definition of minimalism as a musical work created with a minimum of means. Schwarz regards Reich and Glass to be embodiments of modernism, whereas Adams exhibits a postmodern sensibility without a predilection for innovation or systematization. Schwarz observes how Adams synthesizes twentieth-century music, minimalism, and American popular culture into his own art form. The author posits that Adams's early minimalist works already show his intentions of infusing minimalism with the composer's voice and a sense of drama.

88. _____. "Process vs. Intuition in the Recent Works of Steve Reich and John Adams." *American Music* 8, no. 3 (1990): 245–73.

Schwarz examines the development of the early minimalist style. According to the author, Reich's early phase works *Come Out* and *Piano Phase* are created from a singularly mechanized process of development. By the late 1970s, Adams (and Reich) underwent a stylistic change whereby intuitive compositional choices substituted for purer precompositional designs evident in *China Gates* and *Phrygian Gates*. Schwarz elaborates on the structure of *Phrygian Gates* and musical influence stemming from Glass rather than Reich. Following the gate pieces, Schwarz illustrates, through musical analysis, how *Shaker Loops* reveals a more intuitive approach that marks a decisive shift in the composer's musical style. Harmonic processes in *Shaker Loops* are emphasized through contrasts in timbre, texture, dynamics, and figuration, rather than by precompositional structure as seen in the gate works. According to Schwarz, *Shaker Loops* provides the first instance where Adams undermines harmonic stability through oscillations between inner voices or two tonal areas. The author considers compositional developments in *Harmonium* as well, stating that its innovative construction of interlocking canonic lines rearticulates the same pattern in different positions. The musical processes in *Harmonium* and *Grand Pianola Music* resemble Reichian canonic technique, though Schwarz makes an important distinction between Adams and Reich's more recent works: Reich's music has gained complexity over the years yet still clings to the ideal of process music, while Adams composes minimalist music on the surface but rejects the notion of strict processes. Schwarz posits that by the time Adams composed *Harmonielehre* his minimalist origins were relegated to background musical events.

89.   Sheppard, W. Anthony. "The Persistence of Orientalism in the Postmodern
        Operas of Adams and Sellars." In *Representation in Music*, ed. Joshua S. Walden,
        267–86. New York: Cambridge University Press, 2013.

The author investigates the role of orientalist representation in four operatic
works by Adams: the Chinese in *Nixon in China*, Jewish and Palestinian choruses in *The Death of Klinghoffer*, Native Americans in *Doctor Atomic*, and Indian
folktale in *A Flowering Tree*. The author traces the genre of orientalist opera to
the nineteenth century and declares a renewal in Adams's operas, contrary statements by scholars that the genre ended in the postmodern era. The author posits
that staples of orientalist opera performed for today's audiences result in an intertextual influence on the making of new works. Whereas some scholars denote
the emancipation of orientalist signs in postmodern music, Sheppard believes
the position remains utopian, at best. Sheppard attempts to demonstrate Adams
and Sellars's interest in cross-cultural influences and exotic representation of
operatic characters. In *Nixon in China*, Adams sought to avoid using musical
styles that can easily be marked as indigenous Chinese, but Sheppard observes
that his reactionary style does not preclude the opera from functioning in terms
of exoticism. The author highlights some key moments in the opera where the
Chinese characters are portrayed as creating a strong contrast with their American counterparts, focusing on motivic patterns and the music's affective quality. In *The Death of Klinghoffer*, Sheppard posits that the Chorus of the Exiled
Palestinians embodies orientalism through melismatic music, in contrast to the
syllabic writing in the Chorus of Exiled Jews, and is followed by percussive and
primitive music. In *Doctor Atomic*, the author points out that Adams draws on
the *Bhagavad Gita* and incorporates representations of Native Americans, using
exotic lullabies and ritual dances. Adams's approach to exoticism in *A Flowering
Tree* entails the substitution of one cultural reference for another. There are Java-
nese dancers, traditional Indian costumes, references of Balinese *Ketjak*, chorus
texts in Spanish along with wordless choruses, illusions to Mozart's operas, and
a number of references to late Romantic and early twentieth-century composers.
According to Sheppard, Adams's own accounts of the work's conception attest
to an exploration of exotic cultures. Sheppard concludes his study by examining
Adams and Sellars's statements expressing their belief that these operas do not
portray elements of orientalism.

90.   Sholl, Robert. "Searching for the Elusive Obvious: Memory, Forgiveness, Cathar-
        sis, and Transcendence in Contemporary Spiritual Music." In *Contemporary
        Music and Spirituality*, eds. Robert Sholl and Sander van Maas, 229–57. Abing-
        don: Routledge, 2016.

Sholl considers the role of spirituality from the viewpoint of Christian theology
in Adams's *On the Transmigration of Souls* and other works by contemporary
composers Harrison Birtwistle and Brian Ferneyhough. The author posits that
the musical works by these composers share a desire to connect with the divine
source. Sholl engages with Moshe Feldenkrais's concept of the elusive obvious,

which are simple notions that become elusive through habit. The author's central argument states that contemporary spiritual music reveals the elusive obvious. Sholl opines that Adams's work embraces the sanctity or hegemonic power of religion, yet with a malleability that obscures this obvious treatment through the secularization of its language, portrayal of memory, forgiveness, catharsis, and transcendence. Sholl delves into Adams's work, describing aspects of memory, tension, and landscape. According to Sholl, Adams paints an America that cannot recover and cannot remember itself to mourn. Sholl describes how images of presence and absence in aspects such as words, harmony, and textures become a source of spirituality. The author cites how competing polarities—motoric repetition versus harmonic inertia—are dissolved into other possibilities.

91. Taruskin, Richard. "Shall We Change the Subject? A Music Historian Reflects, Part II." *Dissonance* 113 (2011): 36–43.

Taruskin rehashes his argument about the need to control repertoire that could be perceived as insensitive to mourners of tragedy. He reflects on music critics' responses—by Mark Swed and Anthony Tommasini—of Adams's *The Death of Klinghoffer* following the 9/11 terrorist attack. Taruskin opines that critics and musicologists idealized the transgressors in the same way Daniel Barenboim insisted on performing Wagner's music to audiences in Israel. Taruskin refutes the critical responses from musicologists and reasserts his point, noting that present-day conceptions of the role and status of composers are rooted in nineteenth-century notions of idealized transgression and an overemphasis on the individual over collective society.

92. Taylor, Anthony. "John Adams' *Gnarly Buttons*: Context and Analysis, Part 1." *The Clarinet* 37, no. 2 (2010): 72–6.

Taylor's study of Adams's *Gnarly Buttons*, derived from his 2007 dissertation, is published in two separate issues from *The Clarinet*. He begins his introduction of *Gnarly Buttons* by mentioning Adams's anecdote where he expresses his early interest in music from the exposure to his family's Magnavox. He reiterates the history of the commission of this work and its premiere. Adams's opera *The Death of Klinghoffer* was instrumental in creating the composer's musical style that would be suitable for writing his concerto and other works that followed. Adams's stylistic changes result in a faster harmonic rhythm and a blurring of musical lines aided by overt use of counterpoint. To illustrate Adams's post-*Klinghoffer* harmonic language, Taylor provides a musical excerpt from the third movement, which is not duplicated in his dissertation.

93. ____. "John Adams' *Gnarly Buttons*: Context and Analysis, Part 2." *The Clarinet* 38, no. 2 (2011): 66–70.

In this second part of his article, Taylor incorporates some analytical information of *Gnarly Buttons*. The author asserts that some of the prominent compositional tools in the first movement include rhythmic diminution and augmentation, and scalar transformations. Taylor replicates several musical examples from his dissertation that show the development of the opening solo clarinet melody in subsequent measures. In regards to Adams's second movement, Taylor finds musical references from Stravinsky's works and provides examples to illustrate their similarity. Taylor devotes the remainder of his discussion to the third movement, highlighting how Adams's coda is symbolic of his father's illness.

94.   Van Maas, Sander. "The Curvatures of Salvation: Messiaen, Stockhausen, and Adams." In *Contemporary Music and Spirituality*, eds. Robert Sholl and Sander van Maas, 258–74. Abingdon: Routledge, 2016.

Van Maas explores the role of music as a medium of salvation in the works of Messiaen, Stockhausen, and Adams. The author suggests that salvation is related to the curvatures of a sphere, evoking centeredness, binding, and protection. Van Maas's premise is that despite stylistic and religious differences between these composers, their formal emphasis on curvatures serves an organizational role in their principle ideas and compositions. Van Maas discusses a different aspect of salvation for each of these composers: Messiaen and the globalization of salvation; Stockhausen and the deliverance and salvation, facilitated by his own construct of a spherical auditorium; and Adams and the subject of *Doctor Atomic*, which revolves around the creation of the atom bomb, a sphere regarded as the means for self-protection and salvation. Van Maas interprets Adams and Sellars's moral of *Doctor Atomic* as one that shifts salvation from the physical aspect of the bomb towards a focus on how humanity relates to one another and learns to share the planet.

95.   Whittall, Arnold. "Echoes of Old Beliefs: Birtwistle's *Last Supper* and Adams's *El Niño*." *The Musical Times* 143, no. 1881 (2002): 16–26.

Whittall considers Christian symbolism and practices in two contemporary musical works, including Adams's *El Niño*. Whittall purports that Adams's treatment of old beliefs resonates with modern audiences through a revitalization of an old topic presented under a new light. Adams's staged oratorio merges biblical extracts with a contemporary quality through a diversity of texts in different languages. Whittall concurs with Michael Steinberg's opinion that Adams takes a Handelian approach to write his oratorio, noting that the composer does not reserve a single role for each soloist. Whittall asserts that part of Adams's modern treatment entails the depiction of infant Jesus in a non-romanticized fashion, making the extraordinary biblical stories seem ordinary. The author offers a blend of critical reception together with analytical synopsis of various important moments in the oratorio, including Adams's setting of Castellanos's "La anunciación," Gabriela Mistral's "Christmas Star" poem, and Hildegard von Bingen's "O quam preciosa." Whittall shows musical excerpts from *El Niño*, including "Christmas Star" and "A Palm Tree," to highlight their instrumentation, tonality, polyphony, and text-music connections.

5

Select Interviews

TRANSCRIBED AND IN PRINT

96.   Cuno, Jim. "PODCAST: Composer John Adams, Part 1." *The Getty Iris* (May 10, 2017). Accessed May 5, 2019. http://blogs.getty.edu/iris/audio-composer-john-adams-part-1/.

Jim Cuno, president of the J. Paul Getty Trust and an acquaintance of John Adams for over forty years, interviews the composer at the Walt Disney Concert Hall in Los Angeles while the composer was rehearsing a concert version of *Nixon in China*. The two rehash Adams's early upbringing and musical beginnings, speaking about Adams's parents and his first appearance on stage as a performer for a local production of *South Pacific*. Cuno brings up the visit to Harvard that Boulez made while Adams was a student at the university, and Adams reflects on Boulez's approach to music, stating that his style was highly theoretical, with an "intolerant attitude towards creativity and towards style." Concerning the musical environment at Harvard, Adams resented the twelve-tone influence all composers were subjected to during this time. Adams speaks of his interest in electronic music, originating with the first synthesizer the Harvard music department had acquired and leading to Adams's first synthesizer, the Studebaker. Adams discusses a little-known composition he wrote for his master's thesis at Harvard called *Heavy Metal*. The work included readings from William Burroughs's *Naked Lunch*. The recorded interview contains the only known short clip to *Heavy Metal*, and it is assumed Adams must still keep his copy (either in reel format or in digitized form) in his personal library. Another little-known composition the two discuss from the early 1970s is *Lo-Fi*. As the topic of electronic music unfolds, the two speak about another electronic composer who became a good friend of John Adams, named Ingram Marshall.

97.   _____. "PODCAST: Composer John Adams, Part 2." *The Getty Iris* (May 24, 2017). Accessed May 5, 2019. http://blogs.getty.edu/iris/audio-composer-john-adams-part-2/.

The second part of Adams's interview with Cuno picked up from Adams's early career as the composer was beginning to become recognized following the San Francisco Commission and premiere of *Harmonium*. Adams elaborates on the appeal of Dickinson and Donne's poetry in *Harmonium*. Adams characterizes this work as incorporating "*fin-de-siècle* chromatic harmony with the rhythmic and formal procedures of Minimalism." The next topic is the making of *Nixon in China*, from its conception to working out the logistics of the three-person team collaboration. Adams talks at length about *The Death of Klinghoffer* controversy and voices his opinion about the scathing review he received from Leon Klinghoffer's daughters. Speaking of *Doctor Atomic*, Adams divulges the reason that Alice Goodman did not create the libretto for this opera: the Adams-Sellars-Goodman collaboration was always fraught with tension, though the primary reason was that Goodman had become a minister and was preoccupied with sermons and other duties to her church. Adams elaborates on the famous sonnet from the end of the first act in *Doctor Atomic*, "Batter My Heart, Three-Person'd God." This aria is reminiscent of a Baroque passacaglia. Adams's Oppenheimer was remorseful for the creation of the atom bomb, but the real Oppenheimer was proud of his creation and only later in life did he show remorse. The last topic they touch upon is *Girls of the Golden West*, a dramatic work which bears resemblance in name to Puccini's *La Fanciulla del West*.

98.   Daines, Matthew. "An Interview with John Adams." *Opera Quarterly* 13, no. 1 (1996–97): 37–54.

This interview entails a revised transcript from Daines's dissertation. The focus of the interview is on *Nixon in China* and the present and future state of contemporary music. The majority of Adams's responses are more extensive here, while few have been abbreviated without explanation. Comparing the two transcripts shows extensive changes (the author asserts that the earlier version stems from his dissertation) by paraphrasing Adams's words and taking numerous grammatical liberties in the transcription process, as well as rearranging questions. Parts of the interview are omitted in the dissertation transcript, such as the discussion of Richard and Pat Nixon's accounts of Kissinger in their memoirs, which describe him as a womanizer. Readers would receive a more complete picture of the interview by examining both versions since a verbatim transcription of the interview cannot be ascertained from either document.

99.   Darter, Tom. "John Adams the Composer of *Nixon in China* & *The Death of Klinghoffer* Releases His First All-Electronic Album, Created Entirely in His Home MIDI Studio." *Keyboard* (November 1993): 104–5, 107–8, 110, 115–18.

In this keyboard magazine article Darter interviews Adams on composing with the aid of electronics and discusses his all-electronic works, focusing on *Hoodoo Zephyr*, among others. Adams composed the work in his home studio in Berkeley using Musical Instrument Digital Interface (MIDI). Adams reveals the source of inspiration behind the title *Hoodoo Zephyr*, stemming from a combination of desert landscapes, specifically the Valley of Gods, and also the musical influence of the Beatles's *Abbey Road*. Adams speaks on composing with synthesizers and how he began to incorporate electronics into his music, initially in his master's thesis degree, and subsequently in *Nixon in China*, *The Death of Klinghoffer*, and *Hoodoo Zephyr*. Adams provides an inventory of his synthesizers and links those to specific compositions. The composer also discusses the process of transferring his music from the synthesizer to music notation. Adams gives detailed information on the software he has utilized for composition, called Digital Performer (made by *Mark of the Unicorn* or MOTU), as well as how he tweaks the software to alter rhythmic and melodic aspects—drawn from Slonimsky's *Thesaurus*, Scriabin's Prometheus chord, and others. As in other interviews, Adams discusses what attracts him to minimalist music and why he believes it is the most important musical innovation since serialism. Adams is candid about his own musical tastes and how they affect his style of composition. Adams views musical composition as a communicative art form, and for that reason, he is not particularly drawn to the music of Xenakis and Babbitt's scientific approach to musical composition.

100.   Hollingsworth, Leah. "Leila Josefowicz Lends Grit to John Adams' Violin Concerto." *Strings Magazine* 244 (August 2015): 32–6.

Hollingsworth conducts an interview with violinist Leila Josefowicz following her 2015 premiere of Adams's *Scheherazade.2*. Hollingsworth prefaces her interview with a short introduction of Adams's Violin Concerto, describing it as a concerto that explores the subject of inequality and oppression of women. As this concerto was written specifically for Josefowicz, she began to receive sketches of the work as early as 2013 New Year's Eve. Josefowicz, regarded as a proponent of new music, speaks of her experiences performing Adams's three violin concertos. She believes *Scheherazade.2* is closely related to Adams's operatic works as a dramatic symphony for violin and orchestra. Josefowicz describes Adams's orchestral interludes as proportionally larger than the standard violin concerto format, demanding greater emotional output from the orchestra. Josefowicz states she felt a connection to Adams's music and developed a friendship with the composer following her performance of Adams's 1993 Violin Concerto. Josefowicz describes how the learning process of this repertoire demanded her to get in the heroine's character and also channel the voices of women throughout history who have faced oppression. Josefowicz discusses the lack of dramatic closure at the end of the concerto as a metaphor for Scheherazade's struggle and pain that remain in the end.

101.   Jemian, Rebecca and Anne Marie de Zeeuw. "An Interview with John Adams."
        Perspectives of New Music 34, no. 2 (1996): 88–104.

The following interview was conducted on October 24, 1995, at the University of Louisville, after Adams won the Grawemeyer Award for his Violin Concerto (1993). Adams discusses analytical aspects of his work with Rebecca Jemian and Anne Marie de Zeeuw. Adams describes the process of writing his first concerto, from his initial vision of the work as a two-movement concerto (a departure from the traditional model), to a finished product. The work embraces some of the aspects of concerto form, while developing his musical style with a growing emphasis on melodic construction. One of its contributing factors is his incorporation of Nicolas Slonimsky's *Thesaurus of Scales and Melodic Patterns*. A wide range of ideas is discussed in relation to the work: rhythmic aspects and their effect on pulse, compositional influences in the creation of the work, transformational aspects of the music, and tonal closure.

102.   MacMillan, Kyle. "At 70, John Adams Hopes to Preserve an American Influence in Classical Music." *Chicago Symphony Orchestra* (February 25, 2017). Accessed May 5, 2019. https://csosoundsandstories.org/at-70-john-adams-hopes-to-preserve-an-american-influence-in-classical-music/.

MacMillan, a journalist and former writer for the Denver Post's classical music section, speaks with Adams shortly after the composer's 70th birthday. MacMillan inquires about the legacy he has created with a career that spans over 40 years, but the composer prefers not to offer a historical appraisal of his works. Regarding Adams's minimalist style, Adams asserts that his recent works are not composed in a minimalist vein and is puzzled why people refer to him as a minimalist today. Naturally, definitions of minimalism and postminimalism vary among scholars, and I surmise Adams's current style still hangs on to postminimalist traits. One of the factors of Adams's musical style, according to the composer, is an "ethnic American sensibility." Adams speaks of archetypes from American culture that help him to mold his musical works, much like Bartók or Sibelius's own culture stimulated their music. MacMillan proceeds with discussing Adams's upcoming opera: *Girls of the Golden West*. *La Scala* opera house wanted to commission Peter Sellars to write an opera based on Belasco's play, though Sellars and Adams realized that Puccini's libretto constitutes a period piece that fictionalized the gold rush. Their solution was to create a new libretto derived from primary sources. To commemorate his birthday, various orchestras around the world are performing select works from the composer. The Chicago Symphony Orchestra will perform Adams's *Scheherazade.2* under the direction of Esa-Pekka Salonen. Adams describes what it is like to work with Salonen and Leila Josefowicz and to dedicate a work to each of these two accomplished musicians. Other topics MacMillan and Adams touch upon include *The Death of Klinghoffer* controversy, the art of conducting, and being composer-in-residence with the Berlin Philharmonic.

103.   Marshall, Ingram. "John Adams on Conducting Ives." Reprinted in *The John Adams Reader: Essential Writings on an American Composer*, ed. Thomas May, 264–70. Pompton Plains: Amadeus, 2006.

Marshall interviewed Adams on August 1999 in the Sierra Nevada Mountains of California. Marshall begins by asking Adams when he began to be interested in conducting, to which Adams details his first conducting experience during high school. Adams recalls how much he disliked the difficult nature of Ives's Fourth Symphony at first encounter. Today he considers it one of the masterpieces of our time, even describing the final moments of the symphony as sublime. Adams asserts the symphony is rhythmically complex, and to get a sense of its complexities, he entered much of the score into MIDI. Their discussion segues to the music of Nancarrow and his interest in the player piano. Adams is drawn to Ives and Nancarrow for their expansive ability to conceptualize complex rhythms in their works. Adams is also attracted to Ives's music for its pure optimism, whereas he regards works from European composers during this time as more pessimistic. Marshall queries Adams on whether conducting Ives or arrangements of Nancarrow's music influences his musical composition, to which Adams responds affirmatively and elaborates that their rhythmically complex, though accessible approach is a major point in his own musical life.

104.   McCutchan, Ann. "John Adams." In *The Muse That Sings: Composers Speak About the Creative Process*, 63–73. New York City: Oxford University Press, 1999.

For the making of this book, McCutchan interviewed twenty composers, including John Adams in 1997. The author provides Adams's biographical information from his early days as a child to his studies at Harvard, onward to the start of his career in the San Francisco area. McCutchan details other professional achievements by the composer, namely, conducting for major orchestras in the United States and Europe, as well as working as creative chair of the Saint Paul Chamber Orchestra and as music director of the Ojai Festival. One of the topics that seem to separate this interview from others is Adams's revelation of his fascination for Buddhism and the transcendental quest in his music. The composer characterizes his compositional style as having origins in minimalism and over time becoming inclusive of other influences. Adams likens his routine of composing to that of a blue-collar job, honing his craft on a daily basis. For him, every piece poses its own compositional struggles; he might rework the opening after completing the work, as in the introduction to his Chamber Symphony, or he might adapt his musical style to achieve the dramatic aims, as in *I Was Looking at the Ceiling and Then I Saw the Sky*. Adams's approach to composing has changed over the years, initially working closely at a piano, though now relying on MIDI sequencers. Several of his works are the direct result of his music software along with his incorporation of patterns from Slonimsky's *Thesaurus of Scales and Melodic Patterns*, including the second movement of his Chamber Symphony and the Violin Concerto. Another interesting response from Adams addresses his withdrawal of the early version of *Shaker Loops* (and several other unnamed pieces). The composer feels musicians should have the courtesy to respect the composer's wishes and not perform withdrawn works. Adams rejects the musical culture of Milton Babbitt and other composers from the 1950s, for he views them closer to nuclear scientists. Adams sees himself in a continuum of great American composers as a half-vernacular, half-classical composer in the likes of an Ives, Copland, Bernstein, or even Gershwin.

105.   Mijatović, Branislava. "*Ceiling/Sky*: The Music of Double Meanings." *New Sound International Magazine for Music* 12 (1998): 17–21.

Mijatović acquaints readers to John Adams, detailing the composer's East Coast education, followed by his journey and new life in the West Coast, all while highlighting Adams's accolades. Following the introduction, Mijatović provides a transcript from an interview with the composer. The interview touches on the influence of minimalism in Adams, who claims to be working with postminimalist techniques by using the ideas developed by Adams's predecessors in a freer manner that allows for the inclusion of drama. Adams speaks on the influence of Schoenberg and Stravinsky, ultimately regarding Stravinsky more highly for his music's accessibility and pulsation and because Schoenberg suffered from what Adams calls the "prophet complex." Considering unifying themes across his works, Adams divides his works into two broad categories: trickster pieces and more introverted and serious works. Mijatović devotes the latter part of the interview to Adams's first three operas. Adams contrasts *Nixon in China*, a predominantly diatonic, user-friendly opera with a swing-band instrumentation, with *The Death of Klinghoffer*, an opera loosely modeled after Bach's *Passions*, with darker and musically more complex moments, at times atonal. In *I Was Looking at the Ceiling and Then I saw the Sky*, Adams aimed to create a Broadway experience yet sung in its entirety. The interview concludes with a discussion of the defining aspects of postmodernism. Adams's antipathy for the term may result, in part, from its association to early minimalism, a style he no longer seeks to emulate.

106.   Oteri, Frank J. "John Adams: In the Center of American Music." *New Music Box* (January 1, 2001). Accessed May 5, 2019. https://nmbx.newmusicusa.org/john-adams-in-the-center-of-american-music/.

NewMusicBox editor Frank J. Oteri visited Adams at his home on November 11, 2000, for an interview following the completion of the score to *El Niño*. The published transcript touches on the following subjects: success as a composer and cultural relevancy; current cultural landscape; youthful and mature composition; differences in Europe and America; success as an American composer; practical musicianship; setting texts; amplification; religion; a totalist oratorio; beyond experimentation; and technology, chamber music, and the symphony. In composing *El Niño*, Adams stresses setting text with natural inflection and intelligibility. For this reason, melismatic phrasing is uncommon in Adams's vocal music. Adams also discusses amplification of instruments during performances and his interest in composing for the guitar within large works such as *El Niño* and *Naive and Sentimental Music*. Adams offers his thoughts on one of his electronic works that has not received much attention, *Hoodoo Zephyr*, and the composer gives his electronic composition high praise. The conversation moves to the topic of religion, where Adams expresses his background, current views, and his use of the Gnostic Gospels in *El Niño*.

107.　Porter, Andrew. "*Nixon in China*: John Adams in Conversation." *Tempo* 167 (1988): 25–30.

Porter published a transcription of his 1988 *BBC Radio 3* conversation with John Adams recorded in celebration of the British premiere of *Nixon in China*. Adams discusses the making of the opera from its earliest stages, gathering as much source material as possible—newsreels, documentaries, Nixon's memories, Mao Tse-tung's poetry—to inform his understanding of the characters and learn how to inhabit the real-life protagonists in the composer's own musical world. The bulk of the interview explores the depiction of President Richard Nixon, First Lady Pat Nixon, and Chairman Mao Tse-tung. Some critics believed that the opera did not paint Richard Nixon with a realistic tone as a mendacious man capable of great evil. Adams responded that he wanted to highlight the complexities of Nixon in a different way, by displaying his sense of superiority over China and his cruelty to Pat Nixon in their relationship.

108.　Schnabel, Tom. "John Adams." In *Stolen Moments: Conversations with Contemporary Musicians*, 3–6. Los Angeles: Acrobat Books, 1998.

Schnabel furnishes a transcript from a brief interview with Adams. The two discuss Adams's upbringing and musical background. Schnabel queries Adams on the state of modernist music during the inception of minimalist music. Adams favors modes of musical expression that are not overly cerebral in conception and is optimistic that avant-garde styles are waning due to the reemergence of nineteenth-century ideals for human psychological and spiritual values. Speaking on the subject of musical influences, Adams maintains his musical tastes are promiscuous and associates his style as an American aural experience.

109.　Sheffer, Jonathan. "Conversation with John Adams." In *Perceptible Processes: Minimalism and the Baroque*, ed. Claudia Swan, 76–82. New York: Eos Music, 1997.

Sheffer questions Adams on being labeled a minimalist, and Adams responds that the term can be useful yet often too broad in precision. Adams traces the genesis of the musical style, pointing to Riley's *In C* among the earliest examples of the minimalist genre. Adams elaborates on the development of the style and likens it to the growth of living organisms. The composer reflects on the purity of the early style and the way his early works contrasted markedly from the strict and impersonal processes of works from this period. Later, Adams reflects on the role of *Nixon in China* within his oeuvre, discussing notions of nationality and politics, and lauding Alice Goodman's ability to capture Nixon's complex character. To close the interview, Sheffer ponders on the relationship between minimalism and Baroque music, and Adams admits to having a strong affinity for Bach's works.

110.   Smith, Geoff and Nicola Walker Smith. "John Adams Speaks His Mind." *American Record Guide* 58, no. 5 (September–October 1995): 20–4, 47.

This article represents an abridged version of the interview published by Geoff Smith and Nicola Walker Smith in their 1995 book *New Voices: American Composers Talk About Their Music.*

111.   ____. "John Adams." In *New Voices: American Composers Talk About Their Music*, 3–16. Portland: Amadeus, 1995.

Smith and Walker provide information and interviews with twenty-five contemporary composers, including John Adams. Their interview with Adams begins with an exploration of the minimalist style. The key components that characterize this style comprise the repetition of small cells, tonal harmony, and a slow harmonic rhythm. Some of his works referenced in this interview consist of *The Death of Klinghoffer*, *Hoodoo Zephyr*, and *El Dorado*. Adams cites Fred Lerdahl and Ray Jackendoff's *Generative Theory of Tonal Music* (1983) as an influential theoretical book in his development as a composer, affirming ideas about tonality and periodicity he strives for in his music. When asked about intuition in composing (a topic that K. Robert Schwarz has also examined), he likened the idea to the development of stylistic periods that stem from very rational beginnings and reduce their rigor over time. Other topics explored in the interview include the role of the orchestra in contemporary music, finding a balance between acoustic instruments and electronics, and writing operas.

112.   Strickland, Edward. "From *Nixon in China* to Walt Whitman: An Interview with John Adams." *Fanfare* 13, no. 3 (1990): 42, 44, 46, 48, 50, 54, 56, 58, 60, 62.

Strickland conducted this interview shortly after Adams had recorded *The Wound-Dresser* and *Fearful Symmetries* with the Orchestra of St. Luke's. Numerous works are explored during the interview, such as *Shaker Loops*, *Harmonium*, *Grand Pianola Music*, *Fearful Symmetries*, *Nixon in China*, *Eros Piano*, *The Wound-Dresser*, and *The Death of Klinghoffer*. Strickland begins his interview by asking Adams about his professional conducting life. Adams shows interest in conducting Schoenberg's music during this period, which has influenced his 1992 composition Chamber Symphony. In regards to other minimalist composers, Adams admits his affinity for Steve Reich's music for its complexity and conversely his disinterest in Philip Glass's music for its simplicity. The interview continues with a discussion of Adams's studies at Harvard. Adams's response presents a stark contrast to other interviews and his autobiography, stating there was academic laxness, and composers were open to writing in any musical style. Adams reveals having learned orchestration primarily from working with synthesizers. Whereas budding American composers often furthered their studies in Europe, Adams turned to jazz, being influenced most directly by Duke Ellington. He recalls transcribing solos from Charlie Parker, John Coltrane, and Miles Davis. Another noteworthy tidbit of this interview is that Adams acknowledges his Piano Quintet, written with Berg, Schoenberg, and Bartók in mind, as his first mature work. During the time of this interview, the composer had plans to publish the Quintet with some revision, but the project has not come to fruition. Adams discusses other aspects of his music, such as the way he integrates chromatic modulations within a minimalist framework and the development of his style, showing an early focus on harmonic structures and recently a greater preoccupation with polyphonic layers. Near the conclusion of the interview, Strickland asks Adams about religion and whether he believes his religious views seep into his compositions.

113. ____. "John Adams." In *American Composers: Dialogues on Contemporary Music*, 176–94. Bloomington: Indiana University Press, 1991.

Strickland surveys the music of eleven twentieth- and twenty-first-century composers. His chapter on John Adams duplicates, in revised form, his 1990 interview with the composer, which he precedes with a biographical and stylistic glimpse of the life of the composer. Strickland sums up some of the most notable features of Adams's compositions: *American Standard* was written with the influence of Cageian aleatorics; *Phrygian Gates* continued the modal experimentations of first-generation minimalists; *Shaker Loops* combined additive processes with Stravinskian dynamics and dissonance; and *Harmonium* and *Harmonielehre* reflect the influence of Mahler and early Schoenberg, respectively. For Strickland, Copland's call for real American opera has been answered by John Adams.

114. Swed, Mark. "An Interview with John Adams." *Schwann Opus* 6, no. 4 (1995): 6A–7A, 9A, 29A–34A.

This important interview took place before the New York premiere of *I Was Looking at the Ceiling and Then I Saw the Sky* at the Lincoln Center—the work debuted a couple of months earlier in Adams's place of residence: Berkeley, California. Swed catches the readers' attention by claiming Adams has become the Aaron Copland of our time. He continues with a comparison between the two composers, and like other authors who write about John Adams, Swed asserts that the composer's orchestral music is the most widely performed contemporary music today of any composer, with *Short Ride in a Fast Machine* being the most often performed contemporary work. Similar to their treatment of *Shaker Loops*, critics have been less than generous with their remarks about *Ceiling/Sky*. Adams discusses the development of *Shaker Loops* from its original conception for string quartet, initially titled *Wavemaker*, to its mature form for string orchestra. Adams discusses what he called the disastrous beginnings of *Shaker Loops*, and how its revisions afforded him the experience to do the same for *Ceiling/Sky*. In the case of *Ceiling/Sky*, Adams felt that critical information about the characters in the "song play" was missing. On another topic, Adams discusses writing his Violin Concerto, due to his interest in exploring the expressiveness of the violin, as well as experimenting with writing more melodically, which proved instrumental for composing *The Death of Klinghoffer*. Adams also forays into *El Dorado*, a seldom-discussed work in his interviews. He provides detailed information on the construction of the piece as well as its influences. Towards the end of the interview, Adams explores the trickster-versus-serious polarity in his music and equates them to musical traditions: the trickster being American and the serious stemming from European music and composers.

115.   Ueno, Ken. "John Adams on *El Niño* and Vernacular Elements." Reprinted in *The John Adams Reader: Essential Writings on an American Composer*, ed. Thomas May, 183–8. Pompton Plains: Amadeus, 2006.

This article presents a transcript from an interview conducted at the 2001 Ojai Festival, where John Adams was a featured panelist. Ueno inquires about setting Spanish text to music in *El Niño*, to which the composer admits to having reading fluency in Spanish and finding the language appealing for its logical nature and vowel-oriented style. Adams taped a native speaker reading some of the poems in the oratorio to get a sense of the proper flow. The composer describes the collaboration with Peter Sellars, who decided upon the Spanish texts for the oratorio, while the idea of the nativity was suggested by Adams. The poetry by Rosario Castellanos led Adams to come up with a different kind of nativity focused on the role of women in the nativity. The interview switches gears to the subject of conducting music by other composers. Adams believes that exposure to music by other composers instills a deep appreciation for music as varied as the classics, Charles Ives, and Frank Zappa. The last topic Ueno and Adams discuss is the reception of contemporary classical music today.

116.   Varga, Bálint András. "John Adams." In *The Courage of Composers and the Tyranny of Taste: Reflections on New Music*, 20–35. Rochester: University of Rochester Press, 2017.

Varga's chapter on John Adams was drafted from a conversation in Vienna on March 13, 2015. Adams was rehearsing with the Vienna Symphony Orchestra at the time in preparation for a performance of his Chamber Music and the Austrian premiere of *Absolute Jest*. In this interview, Adams voices his frustration with the dominance of pop culture and music because it tends to marginalize other American music, equally representative of the culture, identity, and values shared among its people. Adams speaks on the anxiety of influence today, specifically, how writers portray American composers (and artists in general) as suffering from an inferiority complex vis-à-vis contemporary European tradition. Adams concurs with John Cage that Americans are further away from European traditions and feel less bound to oblige by its parameters, and the composer hypothesizes that European music, beginning with Darmstadt, developed out of a sense of anxiety from composers all too aware of historical precedents. Adams is known to be very candid in discussing his musical influences, and this interview is no exception. In the creation of his opera *Doctor Atomic*, the music of Edgard Varèse served as a model for creating the political atmosphere during the race to create an atomic bomb. For *On The Transmigration of Souls*, a commission he reluctantly accepted, the composer emulates Charles Ives's *Unanswered Question* (Adams elaborates on Ives's influence in detail). The composer concludes that while Ives plays a significant role in his career, someone like Duke

Ellington appeals to him more strongly because he was not fixated on his place in history. More on the topic of influence, Adams is drawn to Aaron Copland's works and he characterizes them as sincere and direct. Adams feels differently about Bernstein because he lost his way as a composer as he gained popular recognition. Adams's views on American music and his own place in history are transparent in the article. Towards the end of the chapter, Varga includes a short commentary by composer Allen Shawn, who is a fellow pupil of Leon Kirchner. Shawn expresses his opinion why Adams has become a huge success in the classical world, and he also provides commentary regarding Adams's thoughts on contemporary music and Leonard Bernstein.

INTERVIEWS AVAILABLE ONLINE

117.   Adams, John. "John Adams: Absolute Jest (2011)." *Boosey.com*. Accessed May 6, 2019. www.boosey.com/podcast/John-Adams-Absolute-Jest/13265.

In this brief video, Adams details the compositional process of *Absolute Jest*. He expresses his love of Beethoven's late string quartets for their *gravitas*, yet he finds the *scherzo* movements equally poignant and energetic in their own manner. Adams sought to recreate the experience of one composer drawing on another in the same vein as Stravinsky remolds Pergolesi's works. Adams dubs *Absolute Jest* the "world's longest scherzo," consisting of a twenty-five-minute collage of musical fragments stemming from Beethoven's works. Adams describes his composition as a trope on Beethoven passing through a hall of mirrors. The composer claims his intent is neither a satire nor a grotesque representation of Beethoven.

118.   Allenby, David. "John Adams Introduces *Girls of the Golden West*" (August 2017). Accessed May 6, 2019. www.boosey.com/cr/news/John-Adams-introduces-Girls-of-the-Golden-West/101032.

David Allenby, who is in charge of publicity and marketing at Boosey & Hawkes Music Publisher, interviews Adams regarding his latest composition, the opera *Girls of the Golden West*. The libretto is compiled by longtime collaborator and director Peter Sellars and organized in two acts. The work is commissioned by the *San Francisco Opera*, *The Dallas Opera*, and the *Dutch National Opera*. The World Premiere took place on November 21, 2017, in the War Memorial Opera House located in San Francisco. Sellars proposed the idea of an opera based on David Belasco's four-act melodrama, which was most famously adapted into an opera by Giacomo Puccini in 1910. Adams claims his opera eschews the romantic fluff from Belasco's play and instead brings contemporary issues to the forefront, including "nativism, racism, opportunistic greed and environmental degradation," as well as a "mad obsession with wealth and material acquisition." The girls in the opera are non-fiction characters whose lives and deaths are notably recorded in history during the gold rush years. Louise Clappe is recognized as the author of the Dame Shirley letters; Josefa Segovia was tragically lynched for killing a drunken miner in self-defense; Lola Montez was an Irish born dancer who gained recognition for her Spanish dancing. Adams approached composing the opera in such a way as to capture some of the feeling from original gold rush songs for their unsentimental quality. Yet Adams's composition in this opera is by no means derivative of the Parlour music from the time; rather, he writes "punchy" music that matches the way people spoke and acted.

119.   Knisely, Richard. "Interview with American Composer John Adams" (August 12, 2014). Accessed May 5, 2019. www.youtube.com/watch?v=2zvVZY3Dhb4.

Ricard Knisely, who was the host of Classical Performances on WGBH radio, provides a comprehensive interview of composer John Adams. Adams talks about his early years living in the East Coast and his desire to explore California after graduating from Harvard. Adams was drawn to Cage's philosophies early in his career, but over time, he lost interest and embraced minimalism for its emphasis on pulsation, tonality, and repetition. Adams notes some European critics regard his music as a form of kitsch. Adams naturally disagrees, and he speaks to high-brow and lowbrow culture and its differences in the U.S. and Europe. Knisely asks Adams about his developing style and composing *Nixon in China*. Their discussion segues to compositional process in Adams's more recent works, including *The Death of Klinghoffer*, *El Niño*, and *My Father Knew Charles Ives*.

120.   Park, Elena. "John Adams Speaks Out About Art in a Time of War." *Andante* (November 2001). Accessed May 14, 2019. https://web.archive.org/web/20050730082733/www.andante.com/article/article.cfm?id=14768.

The classical music website *Andante.com* was permanently shut down on February 1, 2006, although much of the content from their magazine can be accessed using the internet digital archive tool *Wayback Machine* (https://archive.org/web). This article is important in understanding Adams's thoughts about the role of art during a time of war. Moreover, Park's article was published shortly after the cancellation of choruses from *The Death of Klinghoffer* with the Boston Symphony Orchestra in late 2001. Elena Park, former Editor in Chief for *Andante Perspectives*, includes a written transcription of her interview with John Adams. Adams believes that seeking comfort after a time of tragedy is needed, though given enough distance audiences want to be prodded and challenged by classical music. The composer takes a firm stance condemning terrorism, though he believes there are reasons why a terrorist commits these acts, and he feels that American society discourages individuals from examining their causes. Adams speaks of the differences in reception between American and European audiences, the latter of whom were more favorable toward the opera. Adams shares his experience of making his recording of *Klinghoffer* at Abbey Road Studios in London and recalls how audiences were receptive to his reading of Goodman's libretto and hearing his music. Park asks Adams about other performance cancellations during his career, such as *Short Ride in a Fast Machine*, which was programmed the week after Princess Diana died in a car accident, and again, shortly after September 11. The two continue discussing the role of music and whether it can exert influence in the political arena.

121.   Schaefer, John. "#4036: Talking Opera with John Adams, on *Girls of the Golden West*." *New Sounds* (October 16, 2017). Accessed May 6, 2019. www.newsounds. org/story/4036-john-adams-girls-golden-west/.

John Schaefer, who has hosted WNYC's radio series *New Sounds* interviews since 1982, speaks with John Adams on the making of his latest opera, *Girls of the Golden West*. Adams opens the discussion with his timeline for creating a new opera, and his interest in opera as an immersive experience, not only for the listener but also for the composer. Adams's new opera appropriates the title from Puccini's *La Fanciulla del West*; however, Adams remarks he has not seen Puccini's opera in full. Adams notes the differences between the two and feels that his opera is in no way a commentary on Puccini's music. Rather, Adams sought to portray the opera using primary sources from factual people who lived during the gold rush. This includes Dame Shirley's letters, the gold rush diary from Ramón Gil Navarro, who is a Hispanic gold miner, and newspaper accounts of Josefa Segovia. The main female characters in the opera are Dame Shirley, Josefa Segovia, and a fictitious Chinese prostitute that Sellars created for the opera. Schaefer asks Adams about the process of revising opera in all that it entails. Schaefer cites *The Chairman Dances* as an early orchestral piece that was intended for *Nixon in China* yet proved too large to fit within the opera. Another aspect they reflect on is Adams's approach to musical form. Adams claims he interprets opera in free form. In *Girls of the Golden West*, Adams incorporates lyrics from 1850s gold rush songs in a simple musical setting. Adams disdains some aspects of operatic diction—such as rolling the letter R—and prefers the American pronunciation. A compositional aspect of the scoring Adams highlights is the use of sparse instrumentation to parallel the harsh life people from the gold rush era lived. Together with the orchestra, the composer uses an accordion and a guitar, admitting that most people at the time could not afford an accordion, yet the composer wanted to exploit its rustic timbre.

122.   Shilvock, Matthew. "San Francisco Opera: *Girls of the Golden West* by John Adams and Peter Sellars (Discussion Only)." *Works & Process at the Guggenheim* (October 4, 2017). Accessed May 6, 2019. www.youtube.com/watch?v=cFygj4EyVTs.

Matthew Shilvock, who is the San Francisco Opera general director, interviews Adams, Sellars, and set designer David Gropman regarding the creation of *Girls of the Golden West*. Adams narrates a slideshow to illustrate life during the gold rush and feature musical scores of songs from this period, which the collaborators integrated into the opera. Sellars elaborates on the background story and synopsis of the opera. The collaborators touch upon some notable moments of the opera, including Lola's spider dance and the final dramatic moment of the opera, involving the lynching of the female protagonist Josefa Segovia, accompanied by an all-male chorus. David Gropman talks about setting the first opera with moving panoramas, and the scene where the miners cut the giant tree stump.

Overall, the interview presents an informative resource on the perspectives of the collaborators regarding the background of the opera, musical influences, and the moral of the story as it relates to our current political climate.

123.   Smith, Anne W. "John Adams, Peter Sellars and *Girls of the Golden West.*" *Commonwealth Club* (October 30, 2017). Accessed May 6, 2019. www.commonwealthclub. org/events/archive/podcast/john-adams-peter-sellars-and-girls-golden-west.

Ann W. Smith, co-chair of the Commonwealth Club of California, interviews Peter Sellars, renowned librettist and director, and Matthew Shilvock, the general director of the San Francisco Opera, on the conception and development of Adams and Sellars's recent opera *Girls of the Golden West*. Adams is noticeably absent in this interview as he was participating in another promotional interview in preparation for the world premiere of the opera, set for November 21, 2017.

Sellars claims the making of this opera took around four years (two years for the libretto and subsequently another two years for the music). The opera is supported by a typical full-sized orchestra, yet Adams uses an accordion for the first time to simulate the mining experience. Since nearly all of the gold-rush literature was written by men and centers around their lives, Adams and Sellars sought to create a more balanced account and depict the lives of women. The newly composed opera incorporates three interwoven stories of the women during the gold rush period in the 1850s. Sellars talks of larger historical themes and draws an analogy to today's current affairs, such as racial inequality. To this end, Sellars shares some of the related history of California and the difficulties immigrants endured, like the Foreign Miners Tax Law, where non-Caucasians were required to pay a tax to live in California. Racism was commonplace, even expressed by the first governor of California, who had an extermination plan for Native Americans. Sellars notes that *Girls of the Golden West* is not the first opera to portray the gold rush; Wagner's *Der Ring des Nibelungen* stands as its Romantic predecessor.

During the gold rush, there was a surge of culture through music and Shakespearean plays in California, and Sellars discusses the California Miners' Ballads, which have become known throughout the world. Sellars gives insight into the remarkable characters of the opera, such as the Chinese prostitute who overcame great struggles and made a life for herself. Another interwoven story is that of Josefa, who had been accosted by a drunk man and stabbed him in defense. A mob ensued to demand her death and she was hanged. In the opera, this event takes place during the fifth scene of the second act. Sellars recalls that Adams's recreation of this scene was initially one-hundred pages long. Another portion of the opera compiles excerpts from a liberated slave named Frederick Douglass who gave an address in Rochester on 1852 about what the Fourth of July means to a slave. To depict Douglass's speech musically, Adams composed a twelve-minute aria that aims for the same kind of emotional and reflective quality as Copland's American standard *Lincoln Portrait*.

6

Doctoral Dissertations, Master's, and Honors Theses

124. Ackerman, David V. "*Symphony No. 1, Redemption*: A Postmodern Symphony with Preliminary Research and Analysis of Alfred Schnittke's Symphony No. 8." D.M.A. dissertation, University of Northern Colorado, 2004.

Ackerman contextualizes his study of Schnittke's Symphony No. 8 by examining other contemporary symphonies, such as Adams's *Harmonielehre* and his Chamber Symphony. The author provides a general account of each movement from the Chamber Symphony, asserting Adams creates the musical effect of chaos through a plethora of rhythmic gestures, fragmentations, and seemingly independent musical lines. Ackerman's overgeneralized observations on the Chamber Symphony are insufficient and readers would benefit for a lengthier treatment, such as Jacob Kohut's 2016 dissertation on formal structure and compositional methods employed in the Chamber Symphony (see item 159).

125. Alburger, Mark. "Minimalism, Multiculturalism, and the Quest for Legitimacy." Ph.D. dissertation, The Claremont Graduate University, 1995.

Alburger frames the genesis of minimalism as a rebellion against other rebellions perceived as evils: namely, serialism and aleatoric music. The author weaves multicultural influences and philosophies which served as new structural models for the Western composers and their minimalist aesthetic. Alburger addresses Eastern influences in the music of early minimalists Riley and Young, who employed Indian scales and tunings, as well as Eastern practices. Alburger references jazz as a musical crosscurrent that had an impact on minimalist composers. In the case of Adams, Alburger notes he has looked to Duke Ellington as a model for improvisation and orchestration. The author remarks the troubled beginning of the minimalist style and traces criticisms it endured from well-known avant-garde composers who were active during the midpoint of the century. Alburger also notes the few critics who were sympathetic to the budding minimalist style. Following this lengthy discussion of the origins of minimalism, the author explores orchestrational aspects in the music of Glass, Reich, and Adams. The three share a common technique of doubling vocal lines with an instrument, and a second technique of composing arpeggiation-style melodies. Alburger gives an overview of Adams's musical background and early minimalist compositions from *Phrygian Gates* onward. He devotes the most attention to examining the stylistic similarities between Glass's works and Adams's *Nixon in China*, even claiming that the opening of the opera draws from the trial scene in *Einstein on the Beach*. Overall, this dissertation educates readers on the reception history of the minimalist movement while providing a brief survey with annotations of Adams's works without delving into deep analysis. Alburger's dissertation is commendable in its length and treatment given its year of publication.

126.   Atkinson, Sean. "An Analytical Model for the Study of Multimedia Compositions: A Case Study in Minimalist Music." Ph.D. dissertation, Florida State University, 2009.

Atkinson develops an analytical model for examining minimalist multimedia compositions, including works by Steve Reich, Philip Glass, and *Bang on a Can* composers, as well as Adams's opera *Nixon in China*. Atkinson emulates existing analytical tools by Nicholas Cook, who integrates literary concepts from semiotics and metaphor. Atkinson's principal thesis is that nuanced interpretations and subtext are only accessible through close examination of entire multimedia structures. Cook's models are designed to compare and contrast musical and visual domains to discern whether they are complementary in nature. However, according to Atkinson, Cook's models do not address underlying meanings. Moreover, Cook addresses text and narrative only in passing. In order to introduce readers who are unfamiliar with semiotics, Atkinson describes it as the study and interpretation of signs. It entails examining semiotic *signs* and *objects*. The author elaborates further on semiotics by introducing some of the most pertinent concepts, including Leonard Ratner's *musical topics* (which are musical signs), Robert Hatten's notion of *markedness* (understanding meaning through opposition), and Michael Klein's writings on *intertextuality* (the notion of musical or stylistic borrowing and how it affects the meaning of a work).

Atkinson's own model for analysis entails a three-step process: (1) analysis of the surface, (2) resulting semiotic interpretation, and (3) blending meanings from multiple domains into a single deeper exegesis. Atkinson asserts that his analysis of Adams's music incorporates writings by Timothy A. Johnson to elucidate on harmonic content and progression, yet in a broader sense that can incorporate jazz-inspired harmonies. Before delving into *Nixon in China*, Atkinson familiarizes readers with film form and technique. The author delves into two important moments in Adams's opera: Act I, Scene 3 (the dinner scene), and Act II, Scene 2 (the ballet scene). Atkinson tracks musical form and harmonic progression in Chou's aria from Act I, illustrating tritone relationships, clashing polyhar-monies, and chord progressions, which are elucidated with neo-Riemannian music-theoretical models. The author notes that contrasting characters can have musical parallels; for instance, as Nixon discusses American and Chinese rela-tions, Adams incorporates C major and E minor triads, presumably reserving the major key for the West.

Atkinson's analytical model for understanding multimedia is depicted using an equilateral triangle that illustrates different domains that make the opera on each side of the geometric shape: characters' actions, musical setting, and the spoken word. These interpretations provide a window into the subtext behind the characters' interaction and public speeches, in combination with Sellars's staging, character action, and Adams's musical depiction of the events. I suspect that Atkinson's method for analysis of multimedia compositions such as Adams's *Nixon in China* is adaptable to subsequent operas by Adams and other contem-porary operas, in general. Future studies might endeavor to compare Adams's operas in collaboration with Goodman and more recent operas where Sellars and Adams compiled the libretti from primary and secondary documentary sources.

127. Ball, James S. "A Conductor's Guide to Selected Contemporary American Orchestral Compositions." D.M.A. dissertation, University of Missouri-Kansas City, 1992.

Ball discusses a select number of compositions that were commissioned for the *Meet the Composer's* Orchestra Residency Program in 1982. The program pro-vided considerable funding to selected composers for a period of three years as well as additional funds for the rehearsals, performance, and recording of their work. The program was funded by the Rockefeller Foundation, the National Endowment for the Arts, the Hewlett Foundation, the Mary Flagler Cary Chari-table Trust, and the Lila Wallace-Reader's Digest Fund. This residency was pivotal in John Adams's compositional career and helped to place him on an interna-tional platform. Ball's dissertation devotes a chapter to Adams, which contains a brief biography, list of works, specific information about *Harmonielehre*, includ-ing its individual movements, and a discussion of its form and musical style. Ball includes information about Adams's instrumentation and a recording of the work (Elektra/Nonesuch 79115-2, 1985), and clarifies that the score is written in transposed form—an important piece of information that Boosey & Hawkes overlooks in their scores. Ball follows the chapter with quotations by Adams from the liner notes of the original recording. Following a detailed discussion of the musical materials from each movement, Ball offers conducting tips and highlights challenges in the performance of *Harmonielehre*.

128. Barsom, Paul Reed. "Large-Scale Tonal Structure in Selected Orchestral Works of John Adams, 1977–1987." Ph.D. dissertation, University of Rochester, 1998.

Barsom's analysis of the large-scale tonal structure of Adams's works begins with *Phrygian Gates*. The author observes Adams's compositional development, initially employing extensive use of precompositional designs (*Phrygian Gates* cited as an example) and classic additive/subtracting processes, subsequently increasing complexity in harmonic design and a more intuitive approach to writing—other writers such as K. Robert Schwarz have made the same remark. Barsom asserts that there is an increasing tendency in Adams's works to create contrasting formal sections, which invites large-scale analysis. The author's dissertation examines passages from *Grand Pianola Music, Harmonielehre, Harmonium, Tromba Lontana, Short Ride in a Fast Machine,* and *Nixon in China,* devoting the most attention to *Short Ride.* In his characterization of Adams's style, Adams delves into minimalism, new-romanticism, and Western art music. One of the topics Barsom ties in connection to large-scale form is Adams's approach to extending harmonies for extended periods. Barsom utilizes Timothy Johnson's chord preference rules developed for the analysis of Adams's harmonies. Barsom provides a lengthy commentary on Johnson's top-down approach and posits that Johnson's rules are arbitrary and misleading, for they always yield an overriding triad or seventh chord without entertaining the notion of polyharmony. Barsom and Johnson's methods are more complementary than elucidated in this study, both allowing for the possibility of embellishing tones within their respective models. Barsom regards transitional passages as a defining aspect in Adams's conception of form, and to this end, the author asserts that Adams creates tonal ambiguity before arriving at a new formal section. The author's analysis of *Short Ride in a Fast Machine* employs polyharmonies in the middle portion, which create ambiguity that subsides in the final section.

129.   Barton, Thomas. "Music, Place, and the Creation of Cultural Memory: A Study of Benjamin Britten's *War Requiem,* John Adams' *On the Transmigration of Souls,* and Steve Reich's *Different Trains.*" Ph.D. dissertation, University of London, 2011.

Barton's central thesis investigates the relationship between music and places of memory, and their implication for geographical studies of cultural memory. The author explores Adams's *On the Transmigration of Souls,* which the composer himself has described as a memory space. Barton's overarching aim is to find parallels between music and architecture. He poses general questions about the value of approaching music spatially, the relationship between music and architecture, and the role of music in creating a cultural memory. Following the introduction, Barton's second chapter investigates key texts, ideas, and schools of thought that support his approach. The third chapter addresses Barton's methodology, which is rooted in a musicological approach and its relationship to the spatial understanding of culture. Subsequent chapters present Barton's case studies, including Adams's *On the Transmigration of Souls.* According to Barton, Adams sought to create a musical image of majestic European cathedrals and their otherworldly essence. Barton supports Adams's personal evocation, stating that the fundamental nature of this work results in a conglomerate of spatial, ethereal, soulful, contemplative elements. Barton concludes by comparing Adams's *Transmigration* to the 9/11 memorial *Reflecting Absence,* designed by the architect Michael Arad.

130.   Beverly, David Bruce. "John Adams's Opera *The Death of Klinghoffer.*" Ph.D. dissertation, University of Kentucky, 2002.

Beverly offers a musicological and historical approach to *The Death of Klinghoffer*. Beverly purports that an understanding of the treatment of the text can stimulate critical analysis of the opera in regards to its structure, language, and confluence of musical styles. Throughout the dissertation, Beverly uses the notion of the *mosaic* from Marshall McLuhan to examine historical accounts, religious sources, and writings from the captain of the cruise ship, all of which provide fragments of the event. Beverly compiles an extensive bibliography of sources on the *Achille Lauro* hijacking ranging from newspapers and magazines to books and journals.

Beverly includes an interview he conducted with Adams on October 25, 1995. While Adams mentions many of his works during the interview (*Phrygian Gates, Shaker Loops, Harmonium, Nixon in China,* the Violin Concerto, *Fearful Symmetries, The Wound-Dresser, I Was Looking at the Ceiling and Then I Saw the Sky*), the principal topic of their discussion centers on *The Death of Klinghoffer*. Adams provides context for his second opera and a window into its creation, offering compelling reasoning why the opera is not anti-Semitic. The interview touches on a wide variety of topics, such as the nature of Adams's trickster pieces, his gating technique witnessed in works from the 70s and 80s, the "Great Performers" production of *Nixon in China* in Houston, the making of *The Death of Klinghoffer*, his evolving musical style, and more. In addition to his interview, Adams's lecture as recipient of the Grawemeyer Award is transcribed in one of his appendices. Beverly also includes a select discography, arranged chronologically by copyright date of recording. The discography serves as a good introduction of available recordings for the readers, but it features only a portion of all recordings, to date.

131.   Biringer, Claire. "Genre, Narration, and Meditation in the Death of Klinghoffer." Master's thesis, University of Washington, 2015.

In her master's thesis, Biringer revisits the topic of this controversial opera and asserts that part of the reason the opera has been unfairly criticized is its faulty assessment as an opera that ascribes to traditional opera narrative. Another aspect of the opera that led to the controversy pertains to the infamous Rumor scene, which features a mundane and materialistic side to the Rumor family, friends of the Klinghoffers. The Rumor scene, which was eventually removed from the opera, appeared in a pivotal moment of the opera, between the "Chorus of the Exiled Palestinians" and the "Chorus of the Exiled Jews" (Thomas May's *The John Adams Reader* reproduces this portion of the libretto in Appendix A). Biringer goes to great lengths to persuade readers how Adams's opera style draws more prominently from oratorio writing than from operatic tradition by substituting arias, duets, trios, ensembles, and choruses with a series of monologues, seeking to elevate events to a higher place where meditation and reflection are the focus of plot development. Biringer interprets Goodman's libretto and

Adams's musical representation as attempting to reach a higher goal by treating the narrative as an allegory of the struggle between Jews and Palestinians.

Examining Adams's compositional layering technique, Biringer notes that Adams interweaves obbligato vocal lines with instrumental ones in a Bachian style. Furthermore, the contour and rhythmic similarities between vocal and instrumental lines raise the status of instrumental parts to a character-defining role. Biringer's examples illustrate how character formation is musically customized for every personality in the opera. The author's thesis provides detailed accounts of Adams's collaboration with the librettist, Alice Goodman. Biringer's bibliography of sources is particularly thorough in documenting primary materials from Adams and other writers on the topic of this opera.

The second half of her thesis explores some noteworthy musicological topics pertaining to Adams's work: "Chaotic Reflection and the Postmodern Era," an evaluation of the opera in light of postmodern characteristics; "Evenhanded Orientalism," Adams's role reversal in the depiction of orientalism, where the Jewish characters are the focus of orientalism; "Opera on Stage and Screen," a foray into Penny Woolcock's 2003 adaptation of the opera; and "Klinghoffer as Meditation," a reflection on the successes of the opera and thoughts on its future reception.

132.   Brege, Casey Jo. "Reception and Influence of a Postmodernist Opera: John Adams's *Nixon in China*, 1987–2011." Honors Thesis, Butler University, 2011.

Brege examines the critical reception of Adams's *Nixon in China* from its premiere in 1987 to 2011. The first chapter considers the reception of the opera following its world premiere. The author reflects on reasons why the reviews were polarized, touching on aspects of the minimalist style and its use in opera, as well as the mythological—rather than satirical—depiction of Richard Nixon. Another area of criticism entails Adams's seemingly plain musical portrayal of Pat Nixon. Brege disagrees with the critics, stating that the lyrical nature of her melodies distances her from the foregrounded political climate and emphasizes her true character. Brege also explores critics' objections with Kissinger and Madame Mao, concluding that early critics did not grasp the intent of the collaborators and the complexity of the opera. Over the years, reviews of this work have become less divided, as it is now a staple of contemporary opera. The author believes critics' new tone demonstrates a deeper examination and appreciation for Adams's work. Brege elaborates on the reception of the work in the U.S. versus internationally, the latter of which was more welcoming from the beginning. *Nixon in China* reached its pinnacle with its 2011 Metropolitan Opera production. This production canonized the opera as one of the classics.

133.   Burggraff, Nathan Paul. "Music and Religion in a Postmodern Culture: Conceptual Integration in Compositions by Glass, Golijov, and Reich." Ph.D. dissertation, University of Rochester, 2015.

Burggraff's dissertation incorporates a section on Adams's restaging of his dramatic works as a means of comparison to the music of Golijov. The author posits that Adams's oratorios *El Niño* and *The Gospel According to the Other Mary* provide musical examples of restaging religious traditions in a manner that might appeal to contemporary culture. *El Niño* diverges from traditional accounts of the nativity story, with a libretto that draws on both the Bible and secular sources, giving the oratorio an eclectic character in line with a postmodern outlook. Moreover, the oratorio shifts the recounting of the story and the perspective from the female's angle. Adams's companion oratorio *The Gospel According to the Other Mary* refocuses the narrative away from Jesus, making Mary Magdalene the principal character. Burggraff elaborates on other aspects of the retelling of the Passion story with a fresh and postmodern perspective on multiple components of the oratorio, such as the libretto, the portrayal of characters, and the topic of female sexuality.

134.   Burkhardt, Rebecca Louise. "The Development of Style in the Music of John Adams from 1978 to 1989." Ph.D. dissertation, University of Texas at Austin, 1993.

Burkhardt's dissertation represents one of the earliest analytical studies on the music of John Adams. The first portion of the dissertation is devoted to the forefathers of the minimalist musical aesthetic: La Monte Young, Terry Riley, Steve Reich, and Philip Glass. In order to contextualize the music of Adams, the author highlights the innovations of his predecessors. Steve Reich codified specific minimalist techniques such as music phasing. Glass developed a gradual additive process for creating musical textures and utilized cyclic structures of juxtaposed rhythmic units. Adams, who joined the fold a decade after his predecessors, exhibited an eclectic style that seemed uninterested in the rigidity that minimalist purity offered.

Burkhardt examines Adams's works from a ten-year period, including *Phrygian Gates*, *Shaker Loops*, *Harmonium*, *Nixon in China*, and *The Wound-Dresser*. Burkhardt asserts that Adams's compositional style in early works from this period—including *Phrygian Gates* and *Shaker Loops*—depart from traditional minimalist qualities in its use of an additive harmonic process, which she examines using pitch-class graphs that show prolongations of notes, key areas, common tones, and note aggregates. Later works from this period, such as *Nixon in China*, exhibit a further shift away from early minimalism through employing dramatic characters in an operatic style, infusing polychords, and using a quicker harmonic rhythm in the last act of the opera. Additionally, the conception of *bona fide* minimalist melodies can be witnessed during this period. The last work examined, *The Wound-Dresser*, shows a move away from diatonicism and towards chromatic harmonic progressions. This work also steers away from minimalism in its use of orchestral imagery, word painting, greater dissonance, and the exclusion of phrase repetition in slower movements.

135.   Chute, James E. "The Reemergence of Tonality in Contemporary Music as Shown in the Works of David Del Tredici, Joseph Schwantner, and John Adams." D.M.A. dissertation, University of Cincinnati, 1991.

Chute's dissertation focuses on three composers who he believes form part of "The New Romanticism" movement: David Del Tredici, Joseph Schwantner, and John Adams. This new trend expressed music with greater consonance and accessibility. Chute explores model pieces from Adams's early style, including *Shaker Loops*, *Harmonium*, and *The Chairman Dances*, and numerous other works by the composer are mentioned in passing. Compared to avant-garde movements of the twentieth-century era, these works exhibit a return to a tonal system, can project pitch centricity, and are driven by relative stability. Chute traces the musical precedents to "The New Tonality" in three chapters: (1) the triumph of serialism, (2) the adventure of experimentalism, and (3) the return to tonality. The first chapter retells the rise of the dodecaphonic system and elucidates its basic model for composition. Chute's explanation for the development of the new tonality is a reactionary one; namely, dodecaphonic and experimental composers reached a dead end.

In his analyses, Chute details characteristic features of each work using standard harmonic analysis without formalizing a method for segmentation. One of the factors for ascertaining chordal roots relates to low pedal tones; thus, register plays a factor in harmonic analysis. Chute advocates analysis using polyharmonies rather than extended sonorities. One of these common juxtapositions found in *Harmonium*, for instance, entails two minor triads whose roots are a whole step apart. Another interesting facet of Adams's musical style is his use of perfect fifths (or their inversion) as a building block in works such as *Shaker Loops* and *The Chairman Dances*. Chute also provides a reductive analysis of *Shaker Loops*, highlighting large-scale prolongations of dominant-to-tonic cadential patterns. Chute incorporates the notion of modulation from common-practice harmony to discuss connections between sections that retain common tones. In considering the workings of *Harmonium*, Chute takes a different approach to examining its harmonies, using a reductive approach that highlights important harmonic moments with Roman numerals. The author purports that Adams's modulations are gradual, which fails to consider the importance of Adams's *gating* technique. He asserts all of Adams's works are written in a tonal style. Depending on how one defines tonality, one could argue in his favor, although Adams has drastically switched gears since his early years.

136.   Colvard, Daniel David. "Three Works by John Adams." Undergraduate Honors Thesis, Dartmouth College, 2004.

Before writing his honors thesis, Colvard was an intern with Adams's music publisher *Boosey & Hawkes*. His time with the publisher gave him a unique opportunity to interview the composer on several occasions. The first interview took place on 9 February 2004, when Adams was serving as conductor in residence at Carney Hall. A second interview occurred on 12 March 2004 at the composer's home. Another person Colvard interviewed for this thesis is Tracy Silverman, who performed the solo electric violin for the premiere of Adams's *The Dharma at Big Sur*, a work written to commemorate the opening of the Walt Disney Concert Hall in Los Angeles. The interview transcripts are essential to scholars exploring Adams's *On the Transmigration of Souls, My Father Knew Charles Ives,* and *The Dharma at Big Sur.*

Colvard notes that the timeline in which Adams composed these three large orchestral works in the span of twenty-one months forms his most prolific compositional period. The background to Adams's *On the Transmigration of Souls* has been documented in other sources and interviews with the composer. It is known that Adams turned to Ives's *The Unanswered Question* as a model for writing his own work, though not as an organizational model, but rather, in the words of Adams, for its "transcendental sense of humanity which . . . is a kind of American version of what Schiller is getting at in 'Ode to Joy.'" Adams's work also hearkens back to musical elements ingrained in his *Harmonium* setting of Dickinson's *Wild Nights.* In *Transmigration,* Adams attempts to intimate the experience of an old cathedral, though not only in affect: sound designer Mark Grey set up fifty speakers throughout Avery Fischer Hall to evoke the right tone for the work. Colvard alludes to the form of the piece, stating that it is organized by the spoken word. The author creates a graph that highlights the dynamic profile and "blocks of temperament" throughout the work. The blocks serve as organizing units that develop throughout the work. Adams cites sixteenth-century parody masses for his integration of Ives's *Unanswered Question*; specifically, the trumpet solo recalls what Ives referred to as "The Perennial Question of Existence." Adams alters Ives's theme in order to end with a minor third; this interval symbolizes the unanswered question from anyone affected by the 9/11 catastrophe. Colvard explains musical sonorities in triadic terms, yet it might prove valuable to explore whether issues of tonal prolongation play a strong factor in this work, and what connotations tonal organization carries in the context of the tragedy. He purports that a technique of *distortion* (through orchestral layering and coloration) is essential to Adams's work. Colvard examines orchestral layering as well as musical quotations as they relate to Ives's Fourth Symphony.

The last chapter is devoted to Adams's *The Dharma at Big Sur.* Initially the work was meant to include passages from *Big Sur* by Jack Kerouac, but gradually Adams moved away from his initial conception and elected to write for electric violin and orchestra. A little-known fact concerning inspiration for the work is that Adams was immersed in the music of an Iranian composer named Kayhan Kalhor. Later portions of Adams's *Dharma* were composed recording Tracy Silverman's improvisations over an orchestral part drafted using MIDI. Adams opts for an archaic tuning system for this work, just intonation, which is influenced by Lou Harrison's music, who preferred the purity of intervals using this tuning system. Colvard notes that Adams's instrumentation was the result of using instruments that could play in just intonation with ease and allow for the use of microtones. Colvard elucidates the modal orientation of the work stemming from a faux raga feel inspired by another minimalist composer, Terry Riley. In sum, Colvard's thesis details some of the larger topics of these three recent works, an important step in understanding Adams's style. Future investigations of these works would illuminate theoretical aspects of the music in closer detail.

137.　Conway, Eoin. "Ur-Motifs in the Piano Works of John Adams." Master's thesis, Royal Irish Academy of Music, 2016.

Conway expands his 2009 article into this thesis by exploring elements of Adams's piano music that contribute to his unique sound. These elements can be observed through an empirical study of recurring musical patterns he refers to as *ur-motifs*. In part one, Conway examines prominent ur-motifs in Adams's piano music by focusing on several musical parameters: melodic, textural, harmonic, structural, and pianistic. The section on melodic and textural parameters is organized into four topics: loops, oscillation, pings, and speech imitation. Conway asserts that Adams's technique of creating loops diverges from Glass and Reich's method for repetition. Furthermore, their early minimalist aesthetic of creating repetition as a mantra analogous to Eastern musical influences is far removed from Adams's approach. Oscillations found as early as *Phrygian Gates* make up the most common melodic ur-motif. These create rippling, wavelike textures that normally grow into diatonic clusters. Conway describes pings as textural or melodic motifs made up of a single note or harmony in the highest register for a given passage. The author posits that Adams used the ping technique extensively from 1978–1987. Conway rightly notes that Adams's melodic lines imitate the natural flow of speech. He cites three instances where Adams uses onomatopoeia to create musical themes: *Lollapalooza*, "Put Your Loving Arms Around Me," and *Hallelujah Junction*. Moreover, his melodic writing mimics linguistic norms where speakers drop the pitch at the end of a sentence and raise it to demarcate a question.

In the next section of his thesis, Conway delves into the following harmonic aspects of Adams's music: diatonic clusters; harmonies stacked, interlocked, or offset by fifths; third relationships; gating; and paradigm shifts. The author posits that diatonic clusters blend consonant and dissonant intervals while eschewing norms of tonal harmony. From Adams's *Eros Piano* onwards, harmonies consisting of juxtaposed fifths became part of his style—resulting from Toru Takemitsu's influence. Conway's writing on Adams's gating technique is inaccurately applied for select chordal changes rather than abrupt modulations that occur between formal sections. Conway's structural ur-motifs entail mutation and delayed bass. His usage of mutation pertains to the gradual change of repetitive patterns. Looking at Adams's mutations in *Road Movies* elucidates the development of his opening musical idea. In the final part of his study, Conway provides a detailed motivic analysis of Adams's *Hallelujah Junction*. In his thesis, Conway presents a painstaking number of compositional techniques as a practical guide for musicians, in a manner reminiscent to Jamey Abersold's instructional jazz books.

138.　Cotter, Alice Miller. "Sketches of Grief: Genesis, Compositional Practice, and Revision in the Operas of John Adams." Ph.D. dissertation, Princeton University, 2016.

Cotter's dissertation is presently the only study that contains primary sources drawn from Adams's own personal archive. Cotter incorporates select facsimiles of Adams's manuscripts from *Harmonielehre*, *Nixon in China*, *The Chairman*

Dances, *The Death of Klinghoffer*, and *Doctor Atomic*; drafted libretti from *Nixon in China* and *Doctor Atomic*; personal journals, along with a diary dated 1983–1984; and correspondence between Adams and Goodman on *Nixon in China*. The central thesis of Cotter's study highlights the conceptual and ethical problems that surface in *Nixon in China*, *The Death of Klinghoffer*, and *Doctor Atomic* and the solutions created by its collaborators. The author remarks that Adams's approach to expressing musical tragedy differs in each opera by drawing attention to human rights abuses in *Nixon*, terrorism in *Klinghoffer*, or annihilation in *Doctor Atomic*.

Part One, entitled "The 'lost' *Nixon* Sketches: Observations on the Genesis of *Nixon in China*," portrays Adams's compositional period as one where the composer sought to distance himself from academic serialism, drawing on earlier musical experiments from *Harmonielehre* and *The Chairman Dances*. As a precursor to the discussion of this opera, Cotter touches upon numerous subjects, including Adams's freer compositional style following *Shaker Loops*, his meeting with Sellars, and his interest in Jungian psychology. Cotter concurs with Catherine Ann Pellegrino that the sonority designated as [027] using pitch-class set theory is a staple of Adams's music. Cotter subjects this harmonic structure using a top-down analytical approach by looking for repetitions to show organic growth. The methodology of pitch-class set theory might likely yield some interesting findings, yet the importance of [027] is not made evident in the initial sketch to *Harmonielehre* (Figure 1.2), where it only occurs as a subset of a larger sonority. Nevertheless, the author attempts to provide Adams's gradual process from initial sketches to a work's more completed version, as well as draw attention to post-premiere edits in works like *The Chairman Dances*.

Part Two, entitled "The Politics of Revision: Twenty Years of Klinghoffer," details the genesis of this opera and its three extensive revisions over a period of two decades. According to Cotter, the initial production of *Klinghoffer* seemed disconnected between its creative musical setting and the portrayal of the terrorist hijacking. Cotter illustrates how the germinating ideas for the opera stemmed from simple sketches of rhythmic cells devoid of melodic contour. Other sketches feature how Adams allowed the natural flow of the text to be expressed musically, which was a remarkably different approach than in *Nixon in China*. Another model for composing *Klinghoffer* was Schoenberg; this influence surfaces in the opera with the presence of the Austrian woman. After a careful study of the sketches used to draft the premiere version, Cotter devotes attention to the scathing reviews Adams and Goodman received for the opera. Initially, the creators responded defensively, followed by their deletion of the Rumors scene, which then led to further harsh criticism and claims that removing the scene was an admission of guilt. The other revisions alter the Austrian woman and the synthesized instruments from the original score.

Part Three, entitled "Sketches of Grief: The Writing of *Doctor Atomic*," looks at the musical processes that shaped this opera, including Goodman's role as librettist, followed by her resignation from the project, and the subsequent Adams/Sellars libretto drawn verbatim from documentary sources. According to Cotter, Goodman was reluctant to show drafts of her libretto and postponed all submissions, eventually concluding that she found the opera subject to be anti-Semitic. It seems that Goodman's resentment from the harsh criticisms of her libretto from *The Death of Klinghoffer* resurfaced when faced with the task of writing an opera about another Jewish protagonist. Cotter asserts that some of Adams's pencil sketches illustrate early stages in the compositional process, which were combined with computer tools such as the music software called Digital Performer Adams uses for composition. The author explores different stages in the writing process of the celebrated aria, "Batter My Heart," as well as the role of Kitty Oppenheimer and more.

139.   Daines, Matthew Nicholas. "Telling the Truth About *Nixon*: Parody, Cultural Representation, and Gender Politics in John Adams's Opera *Nixon in China*." Ph.D. dissertation, University of California at Davis, 1995.

Daines writes a musicological study of Adams's *Nixon in China*. The first chapters provide an exploration of the composer's music and detailed information on the making of the opera. The next two chapters contain transcripts from Daines's interviews with John Adams and Peter Sellars, dated March 22, 1994, and May 12, 1994, respectively. Chapter 5, titled "Postmodernism, Parody, and the Reagan Era: The Airport and Banquet Scenes of *Nixon in China*," touches on elements of parody in the opera. Many of the conventions from traditional grand opera are subverted: the characters are based on living people, rather than mythical stories, and according to Daines, there is a narrative plot unlike that of a traditional opera. In Chapter 6, titled "Fact, Fiction, and Cultural Representation: The Study Scene and *The Red Detachment of Women*," Daines believes that the collaborators show a deep understanding of Chinese culture and their Chinese characters are given a real sense of identity. The collaborators recreate the Cultural Revolution in a complex manner that shuns surface depictions of the Orient from earlier operas, such as Puccini's *Madama Butterfly*. In Chapter 7, titled "Nixon's Women: The Gender Politics of *Nixon in China*," Daines asserts that the opera plots an elaborate trajectory for the development of the female characters by initially maintaining a subordinate role in Act I, and subsequently upsetting those expectations in Act II and thereafter. The result is a portrayal of strong women with great influence. In Chapter 8, titled "Gender Relations, Cultural Representation, and Parody: Act III of *Nixon in China*," Daines ties in these three aspects of his discussion and maintains they are inseparable throughout the opera. In the end, Daines provides appendices with a discography of Adams's works, list of compositions, and performances of *Nixon in China*.

140.   Derfler, Brandon Joel. "Process as Problem, Problem as Process: Schoenberg and John Adams." Master's thesis, University of North Carolina at Chapel Hill, 1998.

Derfler's examination of Schoenberg's influence on Adams is commendable for a master's thesis. Derfler begins with the premise that Adams abandons his minimalist roots early in his compositional career in favor of a motivic and organic approach to composition. The author asserts that Adams's impetus for steering away from pure minimalism is Schoenberg's *Harmonielehre*. According to Derfler, Adams's *Phrygian Gates* constitutes Adams's only minimalist work. Derfler draws parallels between Schoenberg and Adams's instrumentation for numerous works that have a similar chronological timeframe. According to Derfler, Adams's organic approach to composition diverges from the process-driven style of minimalists such as Glass, Reich, and Riley. The distinctions are made clear by the author: process music gives the impression that the music is devoid of agency, whereas organic forms make manifest the composer's voice through contrasting formal sections and the will to shift gears at any point. Derfler speculates that Adams's gating technique stems from Reich's own method of quick modulations prominent in *Music for Mallet Instruments, Voices, and Organ* (1973). Reich's phasing loosely influences Adams's *Shaker Loops*. Looking at another early minimalist work by Adams, Derfler graphs the precompositional building block of "A System of Weights and Measures" from *Phrygian Gates*.

In Chapter 2 Derfler asserts that Adams steered away from composing nondiatonic music during his formative years—*Electric Wake* and the Piano Quintet invalidate this assertion. Despite this minor objection, Derfler is persuasive in drawing connections between Adams and Schoenberg, while incorporating a testament from the composer himself on the subject. The author attempts to employ Schoenberg's ideas on developing variation and organicism as key elements of Adams's minimalist style. Another connection he explores is Schoenberg's *Farben*, and to this goal, Derfler supports his hypothesis by examining several of Adams's early works, notably *Phrygian Gates*. In his analysis of *Harmonium*, Derfler identifies some recurring motifs between movements along with other linking strategies using harmony and key parameters, which, in sum, contribute to the impression of the Germanic tradition of composition. The author discusses another important aspect stemming from Schoenberg's theoretical writings and compositions, known as the concept of fluctuating tonality, which the author equates to a kind of bitonality. Derfler explores Adams's compositions that demonstrate a conflict between two keys a semitone apart, originating as early as *Phrygian Gates*. Another signature trait Derfler discovers pertains to tritone modulations (and secondarily chromatic-mediant progressions) in works from the mid-1980s onwards. Derfler remarks that during this time Adams was influenced by film composers, particularly film scores from James Horner's *Star Trek II* and *III*. Overall, Derfler's thesis offers a cogent interpretation of Adams's works as being influenced most directly by Schoenberg, and he supports his ideas with detailed harmonic analyses (using reductive approaches) and incorporating excerpts by Schoenberg as a means of comparison.

141.   ____. "Single-Voice Transformations: A Model for Parsimonious Voice Leading." Ph.D. dissertation, University of Washington, 2007.

In this music-theoretical dissertation, Derfler explores parsimonious voice-leading connections from post-tonal stylistic periods by Scriabin, Webern, and

Adams, among others. The author creates a theoretical model that examines voice-leading with this aim in mind. This includes the *single semitone transformation*, where a single voice in a chord is transposed by a semitone while otherwise maintaining common tones. Derfler addresses sets of different cardinalities (or sizes) with mathematical operations he calls *split* and *fuse*. It seems to me that this method of analysis is modeled after Timothy Johnson's 1991 *common-tone index* (see item 155).

According to Derfler, John Adams's early diatonic style invites analysis that employs neo-Riemannian tools as well as those described in his dissertation. The author begins his analysis of Adams's works with *China Gates*, highlighting common tones between the four diatonic modes used for the entire piano work. After stressing Adams's preoccupation for maintaining common tones, the author highlights Adams's most pervasive neo-Riemannian operations across various works. In *Grand Pianola Music*, the first movement is governed by *Leittonwechsel* operations, the slow middle movement features *relative* operations more prominently, and the last movement is driven by David Lewin's *slide* operation. Some of the groundwork for understanding *Nixon in China* from Derfler's parsimonious models and their connection to the libretto is discussed. It would be advisable to supplement this author's readings with Timothy Johnson's 2011 book *John Adams's Nixon in China*, which provides neo-Riemannian analyses of the opera (see item 7).

142.   D'Netto, Connor. "Harmonic Progression and Pitch-Centricity in John Adams's *Phrygian Gates*." B.M. thesis, University of Queensland, 2015.

D'Netto offers an examination of harmony and harmonic progression in Adams's *Phrygian Gates*. The author declares his approach, modeled after James Edward Evans's master's thesis, is twofold. First, a micro-level analysis encapsulates textures into vertical structures. Second, a macro-level analysis highlights harmony, voice leading, and prolongation. D'Netto also considers how perceptual ambiguity in the opening section creates conflicting interpretations of tonal centers. D'Netto gives a select literature review consisting primarily of dissertations that examine *Phrygian Gates*. He posits that harmony in *Phrygian Gates* has not been examined in the studies he cites. D'Netto blends Timothy Johnson's analytical tool called the common-tone index with Fred Lerdahl's conditions for musical salience. The result is D'Netto's own chord preference rules that account for arpeggiations, pitch repetition, registral extremities, voice leading, and other aspects to inform the harmonic analysis. D'Netto's macro-level analysis employs the use of Roman numerals yet with uncommon alterations to chord qualities and other modifications from standard harmony. In sum, entertaining the idea of modal ambiguity in Adams's *Phrygian Gates* broadens analytical interpretations for considerations of salience.

143.   Doyle, James Joseph. "*Violetting Through August's End (Or the Sunset in Water, the Carillon-Chime in Square)*: An Original Chamber Opera and a Critical Essay on the Trajectory of American Minimalist Opera." Master's thesis, University of North Texas, 2014.

Doyle's thesis illustrates the trajectory of American minimalist opera from Glass's *Einstein on the Beach* as a point of origin, and subsequently delving into Adams's *Nixon in China* and several other works by Reich and Lang. Doyle supplies a concise biography of Adams's career without using proper citations for each source. The author includes a brief comparison of Glass and Adams's operas for discussion and analysis. Unlike other minimalist composers, Adams infuses his style with neo-Romantic tendencies. According to Doyle, the rising scalar motion in the opening of the opera draws from cyclic structures common to Glass's works. The author highlights salient features of Adams's style of composing that shape the opera, such as the use of canonic structures contained within ostinati, polyrhythms, and polymeters. Adams's harmonic palette is described as tonal, triadic, and consonant, bearing some markings to Reich's style. Doyle observes that Adams's vocal textures are more traditional in character and often recall the style of classic opera. He illustrates several examples of these vocal lines, such as the "News" aria, which resembles Rossini's music, and Mao's spirit of heroism, which bears traces to Wagner's Siegfried. Doyle references Timothy Johnson's *John Adams's Nixon in China* to discuss Adams's harmonic progressions based on root motion by thirds and to discuss principles of neo-Riemannian harmony. Following the short study of Glass and Adams, the author uses these two composers as pillars of the minimalist style to gain a perspective of the development of minimalism in the twenty-first century.

144. Eaton, Rebecca Marie Doran. "Unheard Minimalisms: The Functions of the Minimalist Technique in Film Scores." Ph.D. dissertation, University of Texas at Austin, 2008.

Eaton's dissertation examines minimalism in film music. Eaton begins with an overview, asserting that as early as the 1960s and 70s, minimalism was integrated into short films, experimental films, and documentaries. Eaton describes various ways minimalism is incorporated in film music to provide musical evocations of machines, aliens, a mathematical genius, cultural alterity, and dystopia. Although there is little discussion specific to John Adams, Eaton graphically illustrates a chronological inventory of minimalism in numerous films along with their associated minimalist composers. Many of the referenced films that contain one or more works attributable to Adams have not been cited by other authors: *Tartuffee*, *The Cabinet of Dr. Ramirez*, *The 20th Century: An/The American Tapestry*, and *L'Ora di Religione*. Most recently, the 2009 Italian film nominated for the Golden Globe Awards *I am Love* introduces a wide range of Adams's previously released works.

145. Ebright, Ryan Scott. "Echoes of the Avant-Garde in American Minimalist Opera." Ph.D. dissertation, University of North Carolina at Chapel Hill, 2014.

Musicologist Ebright offers a critical history of minimalist opera using three case studies: Glass's *Satyagraha* (1980), Reich's *The Cave* (1993), and Adams's *Doctor Atomic* (2005). The first portion of his dissertation traces the roots of these operas and views their connection as a byproduct of collaborations between these three minimalist composers during their early careers. Ebright purports that the emergence and development of minimalist opera owes its aesthetic to the early minimalist style. The author believes that Adams's connections to post-war American avant-garde are largely overlooked in the literature. Because these three operas were written long after the genesis of minimalism, the author considers them less aesthetically pure and refers to them as postminimalist. Glass's opera *Einstein of the Beach* was a turning point that helped brand minimalism as the leading musical style of the time. Moreover, Ebright believes Glass's *Einstein* is a paradigmatic work by which other innovative American operas are measured, including those of John Adams.

The next portion considers how narrative and technological modes of communication—and technological anxiety in the case of *Doctor Atomic*— shape the relationship between the listener and performer. Ebright documents a timeline for the creation of *Doctor Atomic* from its inception. In 1999, Pamela Rosenberg, the director of the San Francisco Opera, conceived the idea of writing an opera on the life of J. Robert Oppenheimer and the making of the atom bomb. Initially, Adams rejected the idea of an opera on this subject, but by February 2002, he committed to composing the opera. Ebright inserts Rosenberg's earliest proposed synopsis of the opera from July 2002 in an appendix. This account seems to contradict Adams's assertion in his autobiography that he accepted the subject matter of this new opera almost immediately. Following Goodman's untimely withdrawal from the project, Adams persuaded Sellars to assemble a libretto from various prose and poetic sources. According to Ebright, Adams zooms in on the hours leading up to the explosion in such a way that slows down a sense of time in the opera to match the external passage of time. Ebright concurs with the findings from Yayoi Uno Everett's 2012 study, which purports that Adams's *Doctor Atomic* gradually slows down time as experienced through the plotline (see item 35). Ebright asserts Robert Warren Lintott made the same point several years earlier in his master's thesis (see item 163).

In *Doctor Atomic* and other works by the composer, Adams controls the soundscape by live-mixing amplified singers, instruments, and digital sounds. To accomplish suitable amplification, Adams has involved the sound designer Mark Grey in the production of his works since the early 1990s. According to Ebright, electronic amplification has both musical and dramaturgical ramifications; musically, microphones balance the orchestra with voice, and dramaturgically, it gives Sellars freedom in choreography—Sellars is free to stage performers to sing toward the stage wings, ceiling, or back of the stage. Unlike the video operas of Steve Reich, the amplification of Adams's works remains hidden from the audience. In conclusion, Ebright attempts to tie in the three operas under study, stating all three are documentary in nature and together they push the boundaries of opera conventions. Moreover, all three explore questions of American national identity through their themes and subjects.

146.   Ehman, Caroline. "Reimagining Faust in Postmodern Opera." Ph.D. dissertation, University of Rochester, 2013.

Musicologist Ehman explores how contemporary composers adapt the legend of Faust in their postmodern operas; among them is Adams's *Doctor Atomic*. Ehman's dissertation predates Yayoi Uno Everett's lengthier treatment of the opera in her 2015 book *Reconfiguring Myth and Narrative in Contemporary Opera: Osvaldo Golijov, Kaija Saariaho, John Adams, and Tan Dun* (which also discusses the myth of Faust). Ehman cites Alex Ross's interview with Adams where the critic first suggested Oppenheimer was a postmodern embodiment of Goethe's Faust. The first chapter explores the evolution of Faust and its application to the music realm. The second chapter, entitled "Anti-Fausts," gives an operatic portrayal of Faust that paints an unflattering image as being selfish, deluded, and even a dangerous anti-hero. The third chapter, entitled "Faustian Ambivalence," focuses on operas that depict Faust in a more complex and ambiguous manner. Faust is undoubtedly portrayed by Oppenheimer as the principal character of the opera. According to Ehman, Oppenheimer is a complex and conflicted person, who, on the one hand, advances the nuclear bomb project despite objections raised by scientists, and, on the other hand, is regarded as a sensitive individual, burdened by feelings of remorse over the Manhattan Project. These two facets of Oppenheimer's personality, which are treated using contrasting musical styles, intermingle with greater frequency as the opera unfolds. Adams sets Oppenheimer's vocal lines using short, clipped phrases to portray a cold and expressionless scientist. On a polar opposite of the spectrum, Oppenheimer interacts with his wife in a more sensitive and passionate nature. Here, Oppenheimer's vocal lines take on a free-floating quality. Ehman ties in Oppenheimer's dual personas with musical aspects of harmonic progression and analysis of form. As the opera unfolds, Oppenheimer's personalities morph into one where the scientist is no longer disciplined in his thinking and reflects on the ethical implications of his project. The increasing moral conflict leads to the famous aria "Batter My Heart."

147.   Evans, James Edward. "An Examination of the Role of Macro- and Micro-Level Processes in John Adams's *Phrygian Gates*." Master's thesis, Eastern Kentucky University, 2013.

In his master's thesis, Evans attempts to provide a comprehensive analysis of Adams's *Phrygian Gates* using analytical tools that focus on micro and macro levels of structure. Chapter 1 situates Adams's piece within the composer's repertoire and includes a review of the literature. Evans states his aim is to consolidate the interpretations from other scholars—namely, Kyle Fyr, Timothy A. Johnson, K. Robert Schwarz, and Catherine Ann Pellegrino—and present a unified analysis with several levels of structure. In Chapter 2, Evans explores macro levels of structure, considering different interpretations to formal boundaries of the work as either three or four movements. Another factor that influences one's interpretation of structure pertains to the use of modes as they traverse through a circle-of-fifths progression. In Chapter 3, Evans focuses on a micro-level analysis of phrases, motivic content, contour relationships among the musical patterns, and gradual processes characteristic of the minimalist style. The author begins this section by describing features that define a module, a term Evans uses to describe a formal section. Next, Evans elaborates on divisions within modules and on defining phrases in the context of Adams's piece. Afterwards, the author devotes time to the growth of motivic cells, gradual processes as building blocks, and anomalies in the work—the irregularities Evans speaks of entail deviations from strict unfolding processes. Although the subheadings in the third chapter are ordered in a sensible manner, it can often prove difficult to follow the author's line of thought. Further elaboration of phrases, modules, and phasing would help support his arguments.

148.   Fink, Robert Wallace. "'Arrows of Desire': Long-Range Linear Structure and the Transformation of Musical Energy." Ph.D. dissertation, University of California at Berkeley, 1994.

Fink develops a theory of musical mechanism to elucidate linear aspects of minimalist compositions. He examines some of the well-known works from the minimalist repertoire by Glass, Reich, and Adams. Fink points to Adams's penchant for using metaphors to describe his music; specifically, metaphors about machinery. Fink uses feminist music theory, modeled after Susan McClary, to depict Adams's *Harmonielehre* as an expression of potency and climax associated with macho-sexual imagery. The author characterizes Adams's style as having a greater preoccupation for harmonic structures than contrapuntal lines in a conscious effort to distance itself from twelve-tone serialism, pointing to *Harmonielehre* as evidence. One could argue that Adams blurs distinctions between harmony and counterpoint throughout his career: case in point, *China Gates*, as an early work conceived by linear patterns.

Fink distinguishes Adams as the most postmodern minimalist composer for his attention to *referentiality* and his eclectic style. Fink supports his portrayal of Adams by describing postmodern aspects in works such as *Grand Pianola Music*, *Harmonielehre*, and *Nixon in China*. Fink provides analyses of *Shaker Loops* and *Harmonielehre* to illustrate Adams's compositional development. *Shaker Loops* portrays characteristic gestures of minimalism such as repetition, consonance, and a motoric rhythm. In this work, Fink traces the syntactic discourse and conflict between two different modules. He anthropomorphizes motivic patterns from *Harmonielehre*. A sense of victory is achieved if certain notes behave in certain ways. Likewise, failure is perceived if these notes do not resolve upwards to their intended goal. Additionally, Fink examines the long-range linear structure of *Harmonielehre*.

Fink purports that the anti-academic stance of minimalist composers has resulted in a lack of a coherent body of music theory. Moreover, he opines minimalist music "seems to actively repel analysis" (217). Fink completed his dissertation when scholarship of minimalist music was at its infancy. Several significant studies of minimalism (Timothy Johnson and David Schwarz), published prior to Fink's dissertation, do not appear in his study. Fink has expanded many topics from his dissertation in his 2013 publication *Repeating Ourselves: American Minimal Music as Cultural Practice*. One noteworthy thread is the viewpoint that minimalism is an artistic reflection of the American consumer society.

149.   Fyr, Kyle. "Proportion, Temporality, and Performance Issues in Piano Works of John Adams." Ph.D. dissertation, Indiana University, 2011.

Fyr considers performance issues in John Adams's *China Gates* and *Phrygian Gates* for piano solo and *Hallelujah Pianos* for two pianos. Fyr posits that in the absence of traditional signals that influence a listener's perception of musical time, proportional aspects play a prominent role in shaping these pieces. Fyr introduces various approaches to music and temporarily using Schenkerian theory, recent approaches influenced by linguistics and psychology, approaches to temporality in post-tonal music, broader perspectives of musical time, and other theories developed since 1950—including Justin London's writings on rhythm and Christopher Hasty's 1997 *Meter as Rhythm*.

150.   Greenough, Forest Glen. "Progressive Density in John Adams' *Harmonielehre*: A Systematic Analytic Approach, with Original Composition." D.M.A. dissertation, University of Northern Colorado, 2005.

Greenough begins his dissertation with the premise that traditional analysis is inadequate to inform the cooperative systems of tension and release in Adams's compositions. His study aims to quantify music parameters of harmony, dynamics, register, and rhythm in a single analytical system called *progressive density*, which the author equates to a kind of musical tension. The aim of this analytical tool is to explore how Adams achieves unity and contrast within formal sections. Greenough employs point graphs to depict progressive density across long stretches of the work delineated by an overarching formal section as well as the entire movement.

Greenough parses out the individual music parameters in the discussion, beginning with harmony and relative dissonance. The author summarizes Timothy Johnson's chord preference rules as a viable tool for analysis of Adams's harmonies. Greenough describes Adams's harmonies as being tonal without adhering to traditional functional harmony. Concerning the concept of consonance and dissonance, the author ascribes a dissonance value to every interval, a method modeled after Hindemith's organization of intervals. Greenough also measures dynamics in tandem with the Fletcher-Munson curve, which measures sound-pressure levels to account for multiple facets of audibility including dynamics, timbre, and the number of players per part. He illustrates relative sound pressure levels using linear graphs. In the realm of rhythm, the author creates foreground and background categories to identify different configurations typical in *Harmonielehre*. As with other music parameters, Greenough ascribes a numerical value to measure the kind of background or foreground texture—complementary, overlapping, or multiple configurations—under examination.

In his formal analysis of *Harmonielehre*, Greenough observes that the lowest points of density delineate the form of the composition into a tripartite structure. The moments of decreased density also relate the opening and ending formal sections through sharing rhythmic patterns and longer harmonic structures. Greenough also notes that moments of high density are coupled with high dissonance and then followed by a sudden decrease in tension. In sum, Greenough's study takes an interesting approach to elucidate notions of form through density, and while the integration of Timothy Johnson's tool for harmonic analysis is commendable, Greenough's study could be further strengthened by engaging other scholarly writings on the interrelation between density and formal structure.

151.   He, Xian. "Construction of Female Gender Identities in John Adams's Opera *Nixon in China*." Ph.D. dissertation, The Chinese University of Hong Kong, 2018.

Xian He explores the role of principal female characters in Adams's *Nixon in China*, focusing on their oppression and transcendence of that oppression. The author begins with a discussion of Adams's creative process and provides the plot summary for the opera. He draws on feminist studies, Timothy A. Johnson's book on *Nixon in China*, and the work of Matthew Daines, who has published at length about the role of women in *Nixon in China*. Xian He iterates the point that although the two female protagonists are wildly different, their gender identity narratives bear striking analogs. The author contends that Pat Nixon made sacrifices for her husband's career in politics, and Chiang Ch'ing experienced oppression under the rule of Maoist China. Furthermore, He asserts that the two female characters are alienated by their husbands and typify the role of deserted women.

The two women, however, transcend oppression through reverse femininity, which surfaces as seeking to have influence during the political summit. The author elaborates on Adams's trio "Maoettes" as a reflection of waning political rigidity in China. Another aspect centers on Chiang Ch'ing's empowerment following the performance of the political ballet known as *The Red Detachment of Women*. Pat Nixon's role also develops her own individuality in the opera. He's dissertation incorporates musical analysis in the form of harmonic structure and its textual connections of brief musical passages, as well as longer passages that elucidate harmonic prolongation in entire musical numbers such as in Chiang Ch'ing's aria "I am the wife of Mao Tse-tung."

152.   Herring, David Scott. "The Use of Percussion in Selected Chamber Works 1918–1992." D.M.A. dissertation, Northwestern University, 2004.

Herring compiles a repertoire of twentieth-century chamber works that exhibit salient percussion parts. Among the select chamber works, Herring includes Adams's Chamber Symphony. The author asserts that Adams's choice of percussion instruments is reminiscent of vaudeville and jazz. Herring compares

Adams's instrumentation to various twentieth-century forerunners and notes that Adams's absence of percussion instruments of definite pitch presents a departure from most other chamber works throughout the century. Adams's method for notating percussion instruments is conventional, adopting a traditional five-line staff in place of a percussion staff. Herring notes that Adams's percussion parts interact with the polyphonic textures of the work, and the author elaborates on rhythmic features characteristic of Adams's Chamber Symphony, including changing meters, polymeters, hemiolas, and hocket rhythms.

153.   Hunter, Stephen Andrew. "An Annotated Bibliography and Performance Commentary of the Works for Concert Band and Wind Orchestra by Composers Awarded the Pulitzer Prize in Music 1993–2015, and a List of Their Works for Chamber Wind Ensemble." D.M.A. dissertation, University of Southern Mississippi, 2016.

Hunter assembles a resource for concert band and wind orchestra works from recent Pulitzer Prize composers. The target readership for this compilation includes conductors, performers, and educators. A brief biography of each composer is provided, along with a complete list of works for concert band and wind orchestra, paired with a select bibliography and discography. As one of the more recent Pulitzer Prize winners for *On the Transmigration of Souls*, Adams is included in Hunter's compendium. Hunter lists Adams's works composed for concert band or wind orchestra, including *Grand Pianola Music, Chamber Symphony, Gnarly Buttons, Scratchband,* and *Son of Chamber Symphony.* The author provides a more detailed report on *Grand Pianola Music* that contains the following: date of publication and premiere, publisher information, commission, duration, level of performing difficulty, and performance commentary for conductors. Hunter's dissertation also provides information on arrangements of Adams's works by other musicians, which is detailed in one appendix. These works include *The Chairman Dances, Harmonielehre, Lollapalooza,* and *Short Ride in a Fast Machine.* Moreover, the arrangements facilitate performance for non-professional ensembles by transposing the key down and/or adapting rhythmic patterns while maintaining the general feel of the work.

154.   Jemian, Rebecca. "Rhythmic Organization in Works by Elliott Carter, George Crumb, and John Adams: Rhythmic Frameworks, Timepoints, Periodicity, and Alignment." Ph.D. dissertation, Indiana University, Bloomington, 2001.

Jemian examines rhythmic aspects of three twentieth-century works where meter is not an operative system due to their lack of a multi-level hierarchy of pulses, including among them Adams's *Shaker Loops.* She compares the revision of Adams's 1983 version of *Shaker Loops* for string orchestra to its original 1978 modular version for seven strings. The updated version derived out of transcriptions from what Adams felt were some of the better performances of the original. Jemian focuses on two movements, "Shaking and Trembling" and "Hymning Slews," and elaborates on four rhythmic aspects that are independent of a metric context: (1) rhythmic frameworks, (2) timepoints, (3) periodicity, and (4) alignment. Jemian asserts that variable periodicities in the melodic patterns in *Shaker Loops* affect the perception of timepoints, which she describes as "moment[s] of a composition marked audibly or through notation" (45). Periodicity pertains to the recurrence of musical patterns at regular distances. Alignment refers to the interaction of all of these rhythmic processes. The author produces illustrations of rhythmic frameworks common to *Shaker Loops* using a timepoint structure that tracks time signatures, series of audible pulses, and periodicity. Jemian purports that the alignment of new periodic units bears formal ramifications since they coincide with principal sections of each movement. Conversely, a lack of alignment of periodic units aids in the propelling within formal sections. Jemian's musical analysis leads to the conclusion that while "Shaking and Trembling" and "Hymning Slews" both contain rhythmic timepoints and periodicity, they are conceived in distinctive ways to create continuity and articulate formal designs.

155. Johnson, Timothy A. "Harmony in the Music of John Adams: From *Phrygian Gates* to *Nixon in China*." Ph.D. dissertation, State University of New York, Buffalo, 1991.

Johnson is the first scholar to devote a complete dissertation to the analysis of John Adams's music. To date, Johnson's dissertation, along with a study derived therefrom (published as "Harmonic Vocabulary in the Music of John Adams: A Hierarchical Approach" by the *Journal of Music Theory* in 1993), present the most comprehensive theory of harmony in Adams's musical language.

His dissertation contains reference information with historical, biographical and theoretical sources relevant to the study of Adams's works, including *Phrygian Gates*, *Harmonium*, *Common Tones in Simple Time*, *Harmonielehre*, *Tromba Lontana*, and *Nixon in China*. Johnson asserts that *Phrygian Gates* comprises Adams's first mature work and *Nixon in China* represents the culmination of working with the minimalist style. Johnson's opening chapter examines divergent definitions of the term *minimalism*. He elaborates on the troubled history of the term, noting how its detractors have ridiculed the style on grounds of its simplicity. He states that some writers focus on the unfolding process in minimalist works, while others assert the works exhibit a non-referential quality devoid of teleology. Johnson purports a broader definition of the term, as a technique of reduction of materials and repetition, would encompass a larger body of early works. Johnson's literature review reveals the budding state of scholarly research during the early 1990s. A selection from the author's sources includes historical books from music since 1945 as a whole, as well as writings that focus on the pioneers of minimalism, notably Reich and Glass.

In Chapter 2, Johnson develops a hierarchical model called a complex. The complex entails three different levels of structure: (1) chords consisting of tertian triads and sevenths, (2) sonorities, comprising of chords and additional pitch classes, and (3) fields, or a complete diatonic collection plus other prominent pitch classes. Johnson postulates that Adams's harmonies contain roots and the complex examines the interaction between chord tones and non-chord tones. The triads and seventh chords derived from the diatonic scale form the basis of Johnson's theoretical model.

In Chapter 3, Johnson develops the common-tone index, which is a tool designed to elucidate common-tone relationships between two complexes. According to Johnson, Adams regards the retention of common tones as comparable to modulation in tonal music. High retention of common tones in Adams's complex coincides with a modulation to a closely related key in tonal music. The common-tone index generates a numeric value for the number of common tones between chords, sonorities, and complexes. Johnson details four properties resulting from a comparison between the three basic components that comprise two separate complexes. Johnson defines common-tone index classes and derives a list of all possible chord complex combinations for triads and seventh chords.

In Chapter 4, Johnson describes idiomatic chord progressions in Adams's works. The author purports there are seven specific root and quality relationships that stand out in the works under study: (1) 3-shift, (2) 3–7-shift, (3) 5-shift, (4) R-5-shift, (5) cycle, (6) shift-cycle, and (7) cycle-shift. Several of Johnson's progressions maintain all but one common tone while moving a single voice in stepwise motion, a property known as voice-leading parsimony.

The last chapter redefines Schenker's notion of prolongation for minimalist repertoire by acknowledging stasis as having a similar capability as Schenker's structural ascent to a primary tone and descent to achieve tonal closure. Johnson purports that Adams achieves this prolongation across sections and entire pieces by means of common tones between adjacent complexes or by half-step neighboring motion. Lastly, Johnson categorizes three different kinds of prolongational techniques exhibited in Adams's works, which he names (1) active, (2) passive, and (3) mixed.

156.   Kalm, Stephen. "An Annotated Guide to Baritone and Bass Arias from American Operas in the 1980s." D.M.A. dissertation, City University of New York, 2000.

Kalm purports that late-twentieth-century American opera tradition underwent a renaissance in the 1980s. The author's guide accounts for 119 baritone and bass arias during the aforementioned decade. Kalm devotes one of the entries to Adams's *Nixon in* China. The author provides relevant bibliographical information, including the librettist's name, opera producer, premiere date, opening lines of several arias, baritone and bass singers from the first production, score publisher, call number, and available recordings. Kalm also provides commentary on the synopsis, together with interpretative insights and suggestions by the composer. The arias Kalm discusses in his guide comprise of Nixon's "News has a Kind of Mystery" and "Mister Premiere, Distinguished Guests," and Chou En-lai's "Ladies and Gentlemen, Comrades and Friends" and "I Am Old and Cannot Sleep Forever."

157.   Keller, Renee E. "Compositional and Orchestrational Trends in the Orches-
        tral Percussion Section Between the Years of 1960–2009." D.M.A. dissertation,
        Northwestern University, 2013.

Keller examines percussion writing in orchestral works from 1960 to 2009. The
author includes Adams's *The Chairman Dances* and *Naive and Sentimental Music*
in his extensive list of varied works from myriads of composers. Keller provides a
snapshot of the percussion parts that details the following information: number
of players needed; number of individual instruments required for each work;
optional setup diagrams; solo passages; extended techniques; standard percussion, mallet, and Latin battery; performance difficulty level; incorporation of
ethnic instruments; and whether the section operates as a percussion ensemble.
In regards to *The Chairman Dances*, Keller comments on Adams's choice for percussion instruments, asserting that many of the instruments and their effects are
a crossover from the dance band, and as such, they are appropriate for a work
subtitled "Foxtrot for Orchestra." Keller also comments on Adams's procedure
for writing percussion, using doublings throughout, in addition to the rhythm
section. The solo percussion ensemble at the end is used to depict the effect of a
gramophone slowing and stopping. Along with appendices at the end of the dissertation, Keller includes an index whereby readers can look up select orchestral
works from 1960 to 2009 according to specific percussion instruments.

158.   Kessner, Dolly Eugenio. "Structural Coherence in Late Twentieth Century Music:
        The Linear-Extrapolation Paradigm Applied to Four American Piano Composi-
        tions of Diverse Musical Styles (Martino, Rzewski, Crumb, and Adams)." Ph.D.
        dissertation, University of Southern California, 1992.

Kessner introduces Adams's musical style within the context of the early minimalist aesthetic. Kessner remarks minimalism originated as a form of rebellion against avant-garde compositional movements during the mid-twentieth
century—Adams disagrees with this common belief in his autobiography. Kessner examines *Phrygian* Gates, whose title she speculates likely stems from electronics, rather than from Eastern musical influences. The author links *Phrygian
Gates* to Steve Reich's 1968 electronic machine called *The Phase Shifting Pulse
Gate*. Reich's machine provides an electronic counterpoint to vertical sonorities, while Adams's *Phrygian Gates* resulted in an acoustic range of contrapuntal possibilities for vertical sounds. In composing with the Phrygian mode,
Kessner claims that some pitches serve a structural role for Adams. The author
does not reference Timothy Johnson's 1991 dissertation, though the two agree
that the form of *Phrygian Gates* resembles a tripartite structure reminiscent of
the ternary model statement-contrast-return. Kessner subscribes to a human-
ist/psychological approach to analysis as informed by the writings of Leonard
Meyer and Nicholas Cook. Kessner's inquiry on the formal sections of *Phrygian
Gates* focuses on the manner in which individual notes and patterns have the
potential to project perceptual tonics. In this mode of analysis lies her strongest
assertion, that Adams creates ambiguous sections that alternate more between

clear sections, and that Adams incorporates old musical elements (modes) into a twentieth-century style. Kessner incorporates reductive techniques for analysis and provides various graphs that illustrate foreground and middle-ground structures. The author reveals some awareness of the concluding formal structure (which rewinds the music in retrograde motion), yet without referencing the large-scale symmetrical aspects of work I discuss in my 2014 *Tempo* article.

159. Kohut, Jacot. "An Examination of the Formal Structure and Compositional Methods in John Adams's Chamber Symphony." D.M.A. dissertation, George Mason University, 2016.

Kohut posits that the majority of studies on Adams's works target his earlier compositional style from the 1970s and 80s. More recent works, such as the Chamber Symphony, have not received much attention in scholarly writings. In his introduction, Kohut believes that mass production of recordings transformed American musical nationalism into a more eclectic style of composition for Adams. Adams's compositions have a unifying theme that revolves around the American experience, and the assertion that we live in a freer postmodern musical period in history has been seconded by Adams himself. Kohut's keen assessment of Adams's Chamber Symphony as a non-minimalist work that employs minimalist techniques rings true of much of Adams's output. Throughout the dissertation, Kohut portrays Adams's style using a dichotomy between traditionalist, European-derived aesthetic ideals versus minimalist-driven techniques. The author cites Kyle Gann, who identifies distinct traits of the minimalist music, and shows how Adams's compositional style has developed since *Grand Pianola Music* by displaying a harmonic analysis of this earlier work.

In the third chapter, Kohut provides a seventy-page analysis of Adams's Chamber Symphony. Kohut first addresses melodic components of the work using the concept of tension and release through dissonance, as well as the gradual building of melodic patterns through repetition. Kohut finds some serial techniques in the first movement and detects the use of the octatonic scale in the second movement. Kohut's analysis of melodic segments also subjects melodies to phrase analysis by grouping patterns that lead to points of arrival. The author's phrase analysis serves as a prerequisite for finding thematic ideas and formal structure. Kohut clearly outlines formal structure using common terminology reminiscent of tonal form, including formal section, interlude, development, and closing statement. Kohut introduces the notion of symmetry to discuss aspects of Adams's music that rely on symmetrical scales, including the octatonic and whole-tone scales in the bass line from the second movement. Another aspect of the Chamber Symphony that Kohut explores is orchestration. He purports that Adams creates almost seventy unique timbral colors in an attempt to combine instruments in myriad ways. The author elaborates on Adams's treatment of instrument families. In regards to formal structure and transitions, Kohut adopts the term *dovetailing*, modeled from my 2008 dissertation, whereby formal sections overlap to maintain little loss of rhythmic momentum. While the allusion of cartoon music is well documented in Adams's Chamber Symphony, the author finds there are also references of Stravinsky's Octet, and he demonstrates similarities between their use of scalar content and means of development, providing musical examples and charts based on their intervallic structure.

160.   Ladd, Jason Scott. "An Annotated Bibliography of Contemporary Works Programmable by Wind Band and Orchestra." Ph.D. dissertation, Florida State University, 2009.

Ladd remarks that while the repertoire for wind band and orchestra has grown exponentially within the past sixty years, research studies on contemporary music are scant. In his literature review, Ladd explains he compiles data from the *American Symphony Orchestra League National Task Force* and various writers who have examined data on repertoire performed in the United States and abroad. Ladd cites several studies on music reception as well as the performance of contemporary works. One study correlated highly educated audience members with a favorable view of contemporary music. Another study conducted a survey that asked twenty band members to rate over a thousand works for band and orchestra based on artistic quality; among the highest rated works include Adams's *Short Ride in a Fast Machine*. In a preliminary study by Ladd, the author discovered that Adams's works are most often programed by professional orchestras with the largest budgets and doctoral-granting institutions of higher education. Ladd includes an annotated bibliography of Adams's works along with a rating of these works based on their artistic merit as determined by other published studies. Ladd's data on performances from 2003 to 2008 concludes that Adams's *Short Ride in a Fast Machine* was the most widely performed work during these years. Ladd also tracks the number of performances of Adams's other works, including *Tromba Lontana*, *The Chairman Dances*, Chamber Symphony, the Violin Concerto, *Harmonielehre*, and *Naive and Sentimental Music*.

161.   Lankov, Jeff. "The Solo Piano Compositions of John Adams: Style, Analysis, and Performance." Ph.D. dissertation, New York University, 2014.

Pianist Lankov explores Adams's solo piano compositions. His introductory chapters offer a brief history of minimalism and a glimpse of the forefathers of the minimalist aesthetic, including La Monte Young, Terry Riley, Steve Reich, and Philip Glass. To contextualize Adams's piano works, Lankov details the composer's stylistic developments into several stages: compositions predating 1977, the preclassic phase, the classic phase, and the mannerist phase. The preclassic phase, originating with Adams's gate works, consolidated process-driven organization and tonality into his new mature musical language; this phase presents Adams's first cogent expressions in the minimalist style. The classic phase incorporates minimalist techniques but assumes an ancillary role to a freer manner of composition. Representative works begin with *Harmonium* and *Grand Pianola Music* and extend to *The Death of Klinghoffer*. The mannerist phase, which succeeds Adams's second opera, features a greater emphasis on counterpoint and polyphony—these compositional periods model the four periods I outline in my 2008 dissertation.

The author's analysis of *China Gates* resembles my own findings I presented for the 2012 Society for Music Annual Meeting and subsequently published under in *Tempo* 68, no. 268 (2014). Lankov guides pianists on performance aspects of *China Gates*, offering useful advice on projecting the overall structure in performance. Lankov's analysis of *Phrygian Gates* is more original and in keeping with the thought process of preclassic phase pieces by other composers. Lankov evaluates published analyses of *Phrygian Gates* and informs his own findings by using motivic analysis to track note-additive processes and voice-leading graphs in order to illustrate the workings behind Adams's movement "A System of Weights and Measures." Lankov subsequently undertakes an examination of Adams's *American Berserk* (2001). Lankov incorporates thematic analysis by parsing out three kinds of recurring ideas: scherzo motives, a chorale theme, and connective patterns. The author draws parallels between Adams's *American Berserk* and signature ragtime rhythms. Lankov explores the chorale theme using a kind of comparative analysis that vaguely resembles Jean-Jacques Nattiez's paradigmatic analysis. Another approach Lankov investigates in *American Berserk* is Adams's use of Slonimsky's *Thesaurus of Scales and Melodic Patterns*. Overall, this dissertation effectively intertwines music analysis with its performance implications. Lankov's most novel aspect of his study lies in highlighting performance aspects of Adams's little-known piano piece *American Berserk*.

162. Laytart, Carla Elizabeth. "Piano Music Since 1950: A Taxonomy of Style and Sampling of Repertoire." D.M.A. dissertation, University of Kentucky, 1998.

Laytart explores the development of piano music since the 1950s and its implications on teaching more recent piano repertoire. The author considers how Adams's *China Gates* captures the minimalist style yet transforms its stylistic boundaries. Laytart considers Adams's work in her chapter titled "Art Music," which is contrasted with concurrent music and topics such as jazz, musical theater, film scores, new age music, and ragtime. The author examines the historical antecedents of each of these styles and explores the subject of breaking into the popular mainstream through a tripartite relationship between performance, publication, and teaching. According to this author, Adams's contribution to the piano literature comes from creating a continuity of sound while maintaining a uniform level of intensity across gate changes. In her analysis section, Laytart hints at the musical form of *China Gates* and describes key areas and form, yet overlooks its palindromic structure.

163. Lintott, Robert Warren. "The Manipulation of Time Perception in John Adams's *Doctor Atomic*." Master's thesis, University of Maryland, College Park, 2010.

Lintott's master's thesis explores the notion of time perception in Adams's *Doctor Atomic*. Together with *Nixon in China* and *The Death of Klinghoffer*, Lintott characterizes *Doctor Atomic* as Adams's next "CNN opera." Lintott seems unaware of the disparaging connotation this portrayal carries as well as Adams and Sellars's objection to the label as discussed in an interview with Thomas May. In preparation for an examination of *Doctor Atomic*, Lintott introduces several writings on the subject of time perception. The most comprehensive source is Barbara R. Barry's *Musical Time: The Sense of Order*. Barry categorizes four types of time applicable to music: *synthetic* is synonymous to clock time; *analytic* entails specific points within synthetic time; *formal* uses temporal characteristics of one object to classify another, and *empirical* compares an object and a referent to note differences. Another source Lintott draws from is Carolyn Abbate's book *Unsung Voices*. Abbate brings into question notions of past tense listening and repetition as a building block and a perceptual stasis. Other sources include editor Jonathan D. Kramer's *Time in Contemporary Musical Thought* and Thomas Reiner's *Semiotics of Musical Time*, among others.

The first act of the opera, lasting roughly ninety minutes, encompasses nearly a month's time, whereas the second act, which is similar in length to the first, focuses on the twelve hours leading up to the detonation of the atom bomb. During the final scene of the opera, Adams reverses the relationship of clock time to stage time; thus, Adams depicts the final moments in greater detail than elsewhere (Lintott calculates the final scene slows down the second act by 97%). Lintott identifies moments in the libretto that lead to changes in time. Oppenheimer's statement "No! There are no more minutes, no more seconds! Time has disappeared, it is eternity that reigns now!" foreshadows the slowing of time leading up to the countdown—Adams also gradually slows down the tempo in Act II, Scene 4. To conclude his thesis, Lintott explores the impact of staging on perceived time. The author writes that Sellars uses staging in a way that highlights shifts in time in the libretto and music. Props, lighting, and other staging components "inform the audience of the public nature of documentary scenes and the intimacy of poetic scenes, and therefore their temporal placement" (73).

164.   Lo, Wan-Yi. "East Meets West: Stereotyping the East-Asian Female in Operatic Works from 1885 to 2010." D.M.A. dissertation, Arizona State University, 2013.

Lo discusses two common archetypes composers use to depict Asian female characters in opera: the naive yet desirable person representative of Cio-Cio San in Puccini's *Madama Butterfly* and the cold and bloodthirsty archetype Liù from *Turandot*. According to the author, Adams's Madame Mao from *Nixon in China* personifies both archetypes within a single character, giving her role greater richness and depth. Madame Mao is perceived in the opera as an ambitious, rude, and aggressive woman who has great political power. Lo illustrates how Adams musically paints these character traits through dissonance and a high tessitura. The author purports that Madame Mao experiences a transformation by the end of the opera, becoming softer in character. Lo's preliminary study of Adams's opera provides a model for comparison and contextualization for other operas that portray Asian female characters. In addition to Lo's study, Timothy Johnson's 2011 *John Adams's Nixon in China* offers a detailed assessment of Madame Mao and other political figures depicted in the opera (see item 7).

165. Loranger, Jessica Rose. "Cultural Memory and Collectivity in Music from the 1991 Persian Gulf War." Ph.D. dissertation, University of California, Santa Cruz, 2015.

Musicologist Loranger claims that scholarship on the Persian Gulf War has not received the same coverage as Vietnam and post-9/11 wars. In her chapter entitled "Modern Composers React," Loranger examines Adams's artistic response to the war, dramatizing the terrorist cruise ship hijacking that resulted in *The Death of Klinghoffer* and several works by other composers. The author asserts that these compositions by classical-style composers engage with collectivity differently than Gulf War popular music. Loranger notes that Gulf War popular music observes a group identity and finds comfort in camaraderie, whereas modern composers question the moral integrity of the collective. Adams's opera forces listeners to consider the group identity and histories of both Jews and Palestinians. Loranger provides background information, focusing on how the opera was latent with controversy even before its premiere, providing primary sources that corroborate rehearsals were held in secret with the protection of the armed police in fear of bomb threats. She recounts how the conservative critic Samuel Lipman characterized the world premiere in a negative light, consequently setting the tone for the U.S. premiere, in which Leon Klinghoffer's daughters attended anonymously and subsequently wrote a scathing review of the opera. Loranger's assessment of the opera is a sympathetic one, agreeing with the opera's collaborators that the underlying message expresses how both groups have a shared experience of living through exile. However, Loranger emphasizes Palestine's history does not excuse their people's actions in the murder of Leon Klinghoffer.

166. Lowe, Frederick William. "On the Minimalist Divide: An Analysis of John Adams's *Grand Pianola Music*." D.M.A. dissertation, Northwestern University, 2011.

In his analysis of *Grand Pianola Music*, Lowe explores how Adams's adaptation of the minimalist style "transforms his visual inspirations into a musical soundscape" and intertwines with myriad musical styles and cultural influences (11). Lowe discusses the dream image of two limousines morphing into Steinway pianos, which was the source of inspiration for Adams's work. Lowe's dissertation is divided into two main sections. The first section investigates the development of Adams's style and compositions. Within this section, Lowe explores various subjects: the cultural context that shaped Adams's style, family, and musical training and influences, and *Grand Pianola Music* in the context of Adams's earlier works. Adams's biographical information is derived primarily from his 2008 autobiography, *Hallelujah Junction: Composing an American Life*. Lowe surveys Adams's works, starting from *Phrygian Gates*, and relates its harmonic language to *Grand Pianola Music*. *Shaker Loops* influenced *Grand Pianola Music* in its avoidance of generic musical titles and its continued adoption of the minimalist aesthetic. *Common Tones in Simple Time* features a similar orchestration and pastoral pulse to *Grand Pianola Music*. Another noteworthy work is *Harmonium* for its similar harmonic framework and gradual unfolding development.

The second section presents an overview and analysis of *Grand Pianola Music*, along with an exploration of its large-scale form and structural markers that define formal sections and influence harmony. According to Lowe, Adams employs various minimalist techniques in his early works, including repetition, oscillation, sustained harmonies, the use of rhythmic cells, and a unique sense for orchestration. A distinguishing aspect of Adams's postminimalist style is the clear and unashamed borrowing from pre-existing musical styles and composers. Lowe's analysis elucidates noteworthy points about formal structure: phrases are irregular in length to allow for more variation and freedom, and transitional sections are marked by specific musical signals.

Lowe includes two transcripts from interviews with the composer, dated February 24, 2005, and May 18, 2006. Adams asserts that he rarely envisions an entire musical structure before beginning a composition, a fact that may correspond with his recent works, rather than *China Gates*, *Phrygian Gates*, and *Shaker Loops*. Adams acknowledges influence from Ingram Marshall in using a rhythmic delay between the two piano parts. The element of parody evident in *Grand Pianola Music* (and various other works from Adams's oeuvre) stems from a kind of American humor Adams sees in the writings of Mark Twain, H. L. Mencken, and Hunter S. Thompson, and it is also a response to what the composer views as the pretentious avant-garde. Adams admits he no longer composes strictly in the minimalist style, yet he remains interested in minimalist rhetoric. The interview topics steer in the direction of electronics, where Adams confesses he is creating his own kind of *musique concrete* for *On the Transmigration of Souls* and interludes for *Doctor Atomic*. Adams talks about composing with software, primarily Digital Performer; yet for the making of *On the Transmigration of Souls*, he used a program called SimpleCell. In speaking about his operas and revisions of his music, Adams asserts that he rarely does extensive revisions that affect the overall structure. Adams's statement contrasts with Alice Miller Cotter's findings on revisions to *Nixon in China*, *The Death of Klinghoffer*, and *Doctor Atomic* (see item 138). At the end of his study, Lowe includes several useful appendices for his study, such as a detailed list of discrepancies in the conductor's score and individual parts.

167.   Majorins, Sarah Elizabeth. "Music as a Memorial Space: An Analysis of John Adams's *On the Transmigration of Souls* and *Over the Sojourners*: A Cantata Based on Psalm 146." Ph.D. dissertation, University of California, Davis, 2007.

Majorins provides an analysis of Adams's *On the Transmigration of Souls* and explores how the work functions as a memory space. The opening chapters center on describing the musical characteristics of Adams's work. Majorins outlines traits from the work's incipit that are influenced by Adams's minimalist origins: namely, a steady pulse, repeated sonorities, gradually unfolding patterns, and ostinati. The open fifth textures are reminiscent of organum and evoke the image of a cathedral; a sparse orchestration also contributes to the effect of openness. Majorins focuses on the affective qualities that Adams's work portrays by using narrations of missing persons and messages from the victims' families in lieu of a formal libretto. Majorins contrasts Adams's work with René Clausen's musical work *Memorial* (2003), also composed in memory of the terrorist attack.

The author asserts that Adams's work can be partitioned into four sections, and that the musical style does not adhere to a strict tonal or post-tonal system, but rather creates its own harmonic language. In her analysis, Majorins provides charts that show the recurrences of voices speaking missing persons' names and short messages, along with choral passages where various foreground harmonies are linked with choral settings for either sopranos and tenors, children, or children with adults. The manner in which Majorins delineates formal sections appears to be motivated by her own perception, rather than citing other scholars to persuade readers. Later in her study, Majorins examines the nature of Adams's quotation from Charles Ives's *The Unanswered Question*, asserting that it raises a question that Adams's work is ultimately unable to answer. As the work unfolds, Majorins perceives an eruption of sound, which ends the meditative atmosphere and pushes to a final climax that represents hope emerging from sorrow.

168. Maynard, Olivia. "A Linear Approach to John Adams' Recent Works." Master's thesis, University of Southern Mississippi, 2019.

Maynard provides a linear approach to the musical analysis of Adams's post-1991 works, using *Hallelujah Junction* as a case study. Her methodology is broken down into three stages: formal structure, linear structure and salience, and harmonic support. The author develops preference rules for the analysis of Adams's music: textural dovetailing is the primary marker of formal division; harmonic and rhythmic shifts serve as secondary indicators of formal beginnings; harmonic and rhythmic shifts that either disrupt static patterns or are visually highlighted in the score—with double barlines—are tertiary indicators; and formal divisions are most clearly delineated when these rules are used in combination. In the third chapter, the author provides examples of her methodology using excerpts from *Century Rolls* as a precursor to her analysis of *Hallelujah Junction* in the subsequent chapter. Maynard's linear analysis of *Hallelujah Junction* draws from Timothy A. Johnson's chord-preference rules for the study of Adams's harmony, my own concept of musical dovetailing, and her unique approach to determining pitch saliency. The author demonstrates that these different approaches are not mutually exclusive, but rather can be applied in a holistic manner to elucidate linear aspects of Adams's music.

169. Mosher, David R. "Embodied Meaning in John Adams's *El Niño.*" Master's thesis, University of Houston, 2011.

Mosher analyzes *El Niño* using theories from contour analysis, music and embodied meaning, transformational analysis, and semiotics. His main thesis revolves on the way in which musical analysis uncovers stylistic tropes in *El Niño* and projects layers of narrative meaning expressed through the listener's bodily experience of the music and its characters. The opening chapters are devoted to contour theory methodology, citing respective scholars in the areas of linguistics, music perception, and music theory, as well as a perfunctory glance of semiotics and narrative theory as a precursor to his analysis in the following chapter. Mosher purports that Adams uses melodic contour as a form of subtext that either supports, contradicts, or provides a hidden narrative. Mosher integrates contour analysis to illustrate how it reinforces text by depicting the words "the babe leapt in her womb" with an initial descent followed by an unwavering rise. Conversely, another musical passage discussed in this thesis features with a descending contour graph to depict Christ's descent from heaven into the womb of Mary.

Another area of analysis that Mosher uses to clarify harmonic relations is neo-Riemannian theory. Through this form of analysis, Mosher makes associations between the realms of man, Jesus, and God. Mosher includes the classic *parallel, relative,* and *leading-tone exchange* transformations, but also less-common ones, such as *planing* and *lift*. According to the author, the *lift* transformation signifies a new beginning, and the *planing* transformation symbolizes Christ's coming to man. This type of analysis is complementary to Timothy A. Johnson's 2011 book on *Nixon in China* (see item 7). Mosher also emulates Johnson's chord preference rules found in his 1991 dissertation, yet he extends the methodology to individual textures according to their timbre while graphically illustrating their connection. In his conclusion, Mosher notes that his examination of *El Niño* only scratches the surface of this work (an assertion I would concur with) and his underlying goal is to provide a range of analytical tools geared for postminimalist music.

170. Moss, Linell Gray. "The Chorus as Character in Three American Operas of the Late Twentieth Century." D.M.A. dissertation, University of Cincinnati, 1998.

Moss explores the role of chorus as character in three American operas; among them, Adams's *The Death of Klinghoffer*. Moss proceeds with a survey of Adams's compositions and style, focusing mostly on his first two operatic works. The *Klinghoffer* choruses are a significant part of the opera for their length and interactions with soloists, transforming into a character that affects the drama on stage. The choruses ask rhetorical questions (detailed in Moss's work), which impart a function akin to ancient Greek plays, lamenting and illuminating the characters' experiences. The next portion of the author's inquiry expounds tonal centers, harmonic language, prominent rhythmic features, and formal structure of the choruses studied alongside their respective text. The format of recitatives, arias, and choruses laid out by Adams resembles the standard model, Moss explains, but the autonomy of the choruses that are set to texts not directly tied to the opera gives the impression of an oratorio.

171. Palmese, Michael Edward. "John Adams Composing Through Others: Modeling, Innovation, and Recomposition." Ph.D. dissertation, Louisiana State University, 2019.

Musicologist Palmese examines musical borrowing in Adams's works as a means to explore stylistic development. Palmese suggests three ways that Adams borrows from other composers and styles: modeling, innovation, and recomposition. Adams's *modeling* procedure of adopting or mimicking other composers is evident in his early works. In the second chapter, Palmese discusses Adams's relatively unknown works that predate 1977 in connection with compositional modeling, including *Heavy Metal*, "Christian Zeal and Activity" from *American Standard*, *Ktaadn*, and an obscure work Adams composed in 1972 titled *Hockey Seen: A Nightmare in Three Periods and Sudden Death*.

According to Palmese, Adams's larger ensemble works from the 80s exhibit *innovation* through their adoption and development of other musical styles. The third chapter explores innovation via the synthesis of minimalist techniques into larger orchestral works such as *Shaker Loops*, *Common Tones in Simple Time*, and *Harmonium*. Palmese provides transcribed excerpts from *Ktaadn* and *Hockey Seen*. He presents his own analysis of *Shaker Loops* and *Common Tones in Simple Time*, showing the manner in which Adams's gating technique is applied to large ensemble works.

In the late 80s and 90s, Adams's method of *recomposition* is at the forefront of his evolving signature style. Palmese purports that Adams dabbled in orchestrating various works by other composers as a compositional experiment. To this aim, the fourth chapter illustrates how Adams's orchestrations of *Five Songs of Charles Ives* and Debussy's *Le livre de Baudelaire* are fused with minimalist sensibilities, subsequently influencing works like *My Father Knew Charles Ives*. He compares Adams's arrangements to their original source while providing a textural breakdown of musical lines that accounts for lowest and highest registers and oscillating chords. In an appendix, Palmese reproduces a transcript from a 1973 interview with Adams facilitated by American composer Charles Amirkhanian. The two discuss some of Adams's early pieces, including *Heavy Metal*, the Piano Quintet, and *American Standard*. Adams elaborates on the individual movements from *American Standard*, including "Christian Zeal and Activity" and "Sentimentals," the latter of which is a reworking of Duke Ellington's *Sophisticated Lady*.

172. Pellegrino, Catherine Ann. "Formalist Analysis in the Context of Postmodern Aesthetics: The Music of John Adams as a Case Study." Ph.D. dissertation, Yale University, 1999.

Pellegrino demonstrates the utility and limitations of formalist analysis in the works of John Adams ranging from 1977 to 1989. In the opening chapter, Pellegrino shows how Adams's music differs from early minimalism in its lack of rigor and asceticism, which are characteristics commonly associated with modernist music and are a stark contrast to Adams's postmodern style. Her definition of minimalism includes descriptors like simplicity, impersonality, and consistency as substitutes for what other writers characterize as redundancy. Pellegrino travels back to Adams's early works *Phrygian Gates*, *Shaker Loops*, *Common Tones in Simple Time*, *The Chairman Dances*, and *Tromba Lontana* to highlight Adams's style of writing being divergent from Glass and Reich. Compositional traits that distance Adams from the early minimalists are expressive gestures and dramatic climaxes, showing a return to teleology prominent in the pre-modernist Western musical canon. She notes that Adams's early works are devoid of melody. According to Pellegrino, Adams strives to maintain a balance between the simplicity of minimalism and the complexity of serialism. She elaborates on this point by reflecting on Adams's thoughts on composing *Nixon in China*, an important work that helped steer Adams to a newer compositional style. Pellegrino's depiction of Adams's compositional development illustrates a shift toward greater complexity and chromaticism, and to this end, the author points that several recent works appear as aberrations that hearken to the early style, including *El Dorado* and *Hoodoo Zephyr*.

Pellegrino's second chapter lays the groundwork for her approach to formalist analysis. The author argues how recurring pitch collections and motivic transformations inform brief musical passages, but its effect on larger structures is not readily apparent. She observes how nearly all of Adams's works exhibit stratification (a notion most often associated with Stravinsky's music) to varying degrees, a concept defined as two or more layers that form a whole but exhibit independence through timbre, register, and/or rhythmic setting—furthermore, the pitch content of each layer must be independent and not impact other musical layers. Pellegrino illustrates stratification in *Grand Pianola Music*, *Harmonium*, *Harmonielehre*, *Short Ride in a Fast Machine*, *The Chairman Dances*, and *Tromba Lontana*, and concludes that this deductive method of examination reveals more about harmonic structure than does examining composite structures. Pellegrino discusses common harmonic structures in Adams; using pitch-class set theory, she purports the [027] trichord and [0257] tetrachord are two of the most pervasive pitch-class sets in Adams's music ranging from 1977 to 1989. Pellegrino includes detailed harmonic analyses over long spans of music to illustrate transformations of these pitch collections. This method of analysis contrasts with Timothy A. Johnson's analytical tool devised for the examination of Adams's harmonies. In sum, Pellegrino offers an effective model for stratification that is widely applicable to much of Adams's output.

In the third chapter, Pellegrino illustrates stratified analysis to show aspects of closure and its ramifications on formal structure, a topic that the author explores further in her 2002 *Perspectives of New Music* article.

Pellegrino's fourth chapter strives to encapsulate Adams's aesthetic, focusing on nationalism, accessibility, and disunity, the latter being a trait of postmodern music. The author notes that Adams regards himself as the quintessential American composer in his upbringing, his musical outlook, his film influences, and the topics he explores in his compositions. The author speculates that the most profound American influence on Adams's style is jazz and posits Adams distances himself from modernist ideals through his accessible form of expression and his American identity. On the notion of disunity, the author models notable writers, such as Jonathan D. Kramer. Near the end of her dissertation, Pellegrino gives a bullet-point definition of the primary traits of postmodernism as represented in Adams's works.

173. Pirilli, Lydia. "John Adams' *I Was Looking at the Ceiling and Then I Saw the Sky*: Examination of an Earthquake/Romance." Master's thesis, Wichita State University, 2013.

Pirilli's study examines the creation of Adams's *I Was Looking at the Ceiling and Then I Saw the Sky*. In consideration to readers unfamiliar with Adams, Pirilli gives a brief introduction of the composer, using Adams's autobiography as a source for its content. Pirilli describes the collaboration between Adams, Sellars, and the American poet and librettist June Jordan. Jordan's poetry appealed to Adams for its humor, warmth, and eroticism. Pirilli incorporates interview material on Jordan that has not been widely distributed in other writings yet is significant to the context of the libretto. Jordan moved to California from Harlem in 1989, which is when the Loma Prieta earthquake struck close to Berkeley, where she resides. Jordan gives the analogy of personal relationships as being similar in their tumultuous nature to the devastation of an earthquake. Pirilli asserts that their "songplay" seeks to address important social issues, including racial conflict, persecution of immigrants, sexual identity, homophobia, sexual harassment, gender, discrimination, and violence.

The songplay, as the makers of this production, as well as Sarah Cahill and others, refer to its unique genre, premiered in Berkeley, California, in May 1995. While writers like Sarah Cahill and Mark Swed have given the *Ceiling/Sky* favorable reviews, this work has received much negative attention because of its eclectic nature. I wonder whether staging the premiere at UC Berkeley, a considerably smaller venue than usual for Adams's world premieres, contributed to critics' dismissal of the work as trivial in light of his oeuvre. Pirilli adds context to published reviews and discusses Adams's reaction to the reviews. The author notes that although some critics seem to have been overly harsh in their criticisms, Adams's work has enjoyed much popularity in Europe. Pirilli includes a list of national and international performances of the work starting from the year of its premiere to 2012 as well as professional recordings.

Pirilli begins her musical analysis of the introductory piece. While her mode of analysis—grouping musical segments into diatonic modes—seems sensible for Adams's music, little detail is provided on the motivation behind her approach. Readers would benefit from further examination of the music using Timothy Johnson's theoretical tools designed for an understanding of Adams's music from the same perspective. Pirilli mentions an array of musical terms—diatonicism, pandiatonicism, centricity, rhythmic layering, polymeter, quartal harmonies— as a sampling of Adams's techniques, though readers will likely be left wanting more detail.

In the second chapter of her thesis, Pirilli steps back from scalar and key analysis, and takes a broader look at the songplay as a whole. One of the most informative parts of her analysis traces all the songs from *Ceiling/Sky* and categorizes them according to its genre, characters performing, and its notable features. Pirilli observes that while each character sings in a musical theater style at some point, some characters are portrayed with musical genres. David, the preacher, sings in a gospel or jazz style. Leila, the Planned Parenthood counselor, sings gospel and smooth jazz. And Consuelo, the illegal immigrant, sings in a musical theater style that features exotic percussion, sultry guitar melodies, and slow tempi. A closer look at these characters and their musical depictions from the standpoint of semiotics in music, specifically musical topics (the work of Raymond Monelle, Kofi Agawu, Robert Hatten, and so many others), might shed even more light into musical character depictions and interactions between characters.

174.   Prock, Stephan Martin, III. "Reading Between the Lines: Musical and Dramatic Discourse in John Adams's *Nixon in China*." D.M.A. dissertation, Cornell University, 1993.

Prock introduces his study by giving readers an overview of Adams's pre-*Nixon* compositional style. Prock explains that engaging with postmodernism as either a reactionary movement or one of resistance is the key to understanding Adams's music. The author describes Adams as more postmodern than minimalist, elucidating how Adams employs traditional tonal materials in ways that undermine traditional meanings and context. Prock asserts that Adams's *Harmonielehre* features two emerging postmodern tendencies that help define the composer's style: the first is continuous and overtly neo-Romantic and chromatic, while the second, which is explored more fully in *Nixon in China*, is more quirky, parodic, and discontinuous. Prock also looks at Adams's first mature minimal work, *Phrygian Gates*, to claim how Adams works with the confines of minimalism, yet in less rigorous terms. The sense of directional motion in *Phrygian Gates* departs from earlier forms of minimalism experienced by Reich and Glass. Prock notes that in addition to establishing a kind of goal-directed work, Adams creates abrupt changes in rhythm, meter, key, register, texture, articulation, and dynamics to interrupt the achievement of implied goals. Prock also observes these features in *Shaker Loops* and *Grand Pianola Music*.

The basis of Prock's approach to exploring *Nixon in China* stems from the idea that Adams's work is the result of ambiguous play between diverse musical impulses, a conflict between conservative materials and rhetorical gestures that undermine traditional meanings. Furthermore, in some defining moments of the opera, Alice Goodman's libretto, along with Adams's music, blur the sense of reality. Prock delves into the analysis of *Nixon in China* by examining key aspects: first, surface and syntax, focusing on style; and second, quotation and context, noting how larger contexts generate levels of meaning not readily apparent on the surface. The former elucidates Adams's harmonic vocabulary, among other things. Prock asserts that Adams incorporates diatonic and triadic structures while avoiding classical-style harmonic progressions. The author illustrates some of Adams's harmonic progressions and refers to them as common-tone progressions—these chords meet the criteria for voice-leading parsimony discussed in music-theoretical writings. In non-diatonic contexts, Adams adopts the octatonic scale, particularly in rhythmic passages reminiscent of Stravinsky—notable examples appear in Chou En-lai's arias. Other aspects of surface and syntax are explored, including rhythm and texture. In discussing cadential strategies, Prock concocts the term *cadential ellipsis*, whereby traditional cadential strategies are used abruptly to switch directions in the opera. Prock notes unmistakable references to styles of particular composers and gestures common in tonal music. The author refers to indirect quotations as "style quotations," and he asserts that Wagner's style is strongly perceived through *Nixon in China*, showing parallels in *Das Rheingold* and *Götterdämmerung*. Quotations that have referential meanings are also discussed in this section. The final aspect of Prock's study explores blurred temporal boundaries—how we experience space and time, fact and fiction—in Adams's *Nixon*.

175.   Rand, Gary Ellsworth. "Harmony in the First Movement of *Harmonielehre* by John Adams." D.M.A. dissertation, Northwestern University, 2000.

Rand examines the harmonic structure in the first movement of Adams's *Harmonielehre*. His study is organized into three sections. The first section provides an introduction that considers Adams's work in a critical and historical context. Rand's investigation centers on one of the predominant features of *Harmonielehre*. During Adams's early minimalist period, Adams began the compositional process by first sketching harmonic structures before giving attention to rhythmic factors. Rand explores how Adams conceals harmonic progressions within a tonally closed movement that exhibits ternary form.

The second section examines harmonic structure as a fundamental building block in *Harmonielehre*. Specifically, Rand's analysis focuses on sonorities, movement, and modulation techniques. According to Rand, Adams's sonorities comprise triads and seventh chords. Their movement emphasizes common tones that gradually and predominantly transform employing half-step movement. Rand illustrates harmonic structure with a Roman numeral analysis of long stretches from Adams's work. To this aim, Rand's musical excerpts showcase modulations along with their pivot chords, though some are too brief and lack the proper cadential motion for a *bona fide* modulation.

The last section attempts to encapsulate Adams's harmonic style by cataloging notable aspects of chord progressions and highlights Adams's eclectic mix of styles to form his own brand of minimalism. Rand reiterates Timothy Johnson's 1991 dissertation to describe prominent chord progressions using principles of neo-Riemannian theory (see item 155). Rand reveals that irregular resolutions of dominant-seventh chords are pervasive in *Harmonielehre*; they are stylistically reminiscent of harmonic practices from the Romantic era. All these harmonies, in sum, are integrated in a manner akin to pandiatonicism since they are comprised of a diatonic key yet are non-functional, the author notes. Rand incorporates another method for assessing the structural role of harmonies based on the notion of harmonic density from Adams's *Phrygian Gates*. Rand concludes his study with a summary of the varied harmonic techniques evident in *Harmonielehre*, including common-tone connections, polychords, pandiatonicism, irregular chordal resolutions, and harmonic ambiguity.

176.   Ridderbusch, Michael. "Form in the Music of John Adams." D.M.A. dissertation, West Virginia University, 2018.

Ridderbusch contends recent works from Adams's oeuvre defy methods of formalist analysis and demand examination on their own terms. Ridderbusch begins with a sparse literature review, emphasizing the writings of Catherine Ann Pellegrino and K. Robert Schwarz for his own study. The author adopts Pellegrino's notion of formalism as an aesthetic view that values structure, coherence, closure, and unity. Ridderbusch believes formalist analysis is comprehensive and can yield a singular analysis of an entire composition. The author adduces his argument from analysis of Adams's works, contrasting *Phrygian Gates*—as a model for formalist analysis—with recent works, including *Century Rolls* and *Son of Chamber Symphony*. Formalist analysis in *Phrygian Gates* is explored from the perspective of large-scale tonal coherence, symmetry, pattern completion, and the establishment of harmonic areas. In Adams's works that postdate *Phrygian Gates*, examining content and recurrence through association and stratification gives a clearer picture of Adams's compositional principles. The author elaborates Pellegrino's interpretation of *Phrygian Gates*, while contesting key points of her analysis. The author's examination of *Phrygian Gates* illustrates the overall form using charts that illustrate defining characteristics of each section, yet Ridderbusch seems unaware of other published studies on *Phrygian Gates* (see items 81, 128, 134, 147). Ridderbusch embraces *moment form* and *block form* to elucidate how Adams's recent works are considered non-formalist and discontinuous for their absence of a singular organizing principle that motivates the entire work.

The second chapter seeks to find methods of analysis for Adams's works that do not revolve around pattern completion such as Adams's early work *Phrygian Gates*. Ridderbusch names other twentieth-century composers whose music presents a similar discontinuous narrative from an analytical perspective—such as Stravinsky's musical blocks, or Edgard Varèse's unpredictable musical progressions in *Ameriques*. The author derives three typologies of harmonic structure to distinguish tonal formalism, using primary triads, post-tonal formalism, music-theoretical pitch-class sets that relate through transposition and inversion, and post-tonal non-formalism, where harmonic structures develop through motivic growth and purportedly cannot be measured through traditional analytical methods. Yet Ridderbusch's assumption that non-formalist music defies standard analysis is misguided, and his illustration of motivic development in the dissertation's Figure 6 can be elucidated with theoretical tools such as Klumpenhouwer networks (K-nets), to name a few.

Ridderbusch's third chapter examines formal aspects of *Century Rolls* and *Son of Chamber Symphony*. The author's discourse focuses on the interplay between formal expectations of sonata and concerto form and discontinuous thematic content. Ridderbusch describes how discontinuity chips away at the core of sonata form through the lack of thematic development and the absence of thematic return in the recapitulation. Alongside his examination of musical form in *Century Rolls*, the notion of stratification and its ramifications on block form are explored.

177.   Rivera, Luis C. "A Repurposing of Orchestral Chamber Works for the Modern Percussion Ensemble." D.M.A. dissertation, Florida State University, 2012.

The primary aim of Rivera's doctoral thesis is to arrange three works—by Reich, Glass, and Adams—for percussion ensemble. The chosen work for Adams is *Phrygian Gates*. To this end, Rivera begins with an exploration of the minimalist aesthetic and provides supporting information on each of the composers discussed. Rivera includes musical analysis, a discussion on the process of arranging for percussion, and detailed information of his instrumentation and its stage setup. In his analysis, Rivera concisely elucidates key areas considering their modal centers and formal sections of the work. Rivera also explains rhythmic aspects of *Phrygian Gates*, such as written versus perceived meter, the content of repeated motivic patterns and their interaction when both hands are performing displaced patterns of varying lengths. The author purports that Adams's use of the damper pedal often demarcates new phrases. On the topic of instrumentation, Rivera elaborates on percussion instruments most suitable for *Phrygian Gates*—Rivera uses the vibraphone to mimic the sustaining effect of pedaling, though its range is smaller than the piano; therefore, marimbas and bells are included in the ensemble. The author also considers a suitable tempo, decided in part from Adams's original tempo, but also in consideration with playability of percussion instruments.

178.   Robinson, Emily Marie. "Inspirations and Influences: Popular Composition Trends in the Contemporary Clarinet Repertoire (1996–2010)." D.M.A. dissertation, University of Maryland, 2015.

Robinson explores recent works for clarinet repertoire; her selection includes Adams's *Gnarly Buttons*. Robinson cites Adams's anecdote of how *Gnarly Buttons* came to fruition. Following this topic, Robinson gives a description of each of the three movements from *Gnarly Buttons*. In an attempt to situate Adams within the discourse of minimalist composers, Robinson introduces Adams's compositional background and ties in various musical traits from *Gnarly Buttons* to their minimalist origins. Robinson purports that the application of a steady pulse, contemporary diatonicism, evenness of dynamics, lack of emotionalism, and avoidance of linear formal design are defining traits in *Gnarly Buttons* that stem from the minimalist style—other authors would contest this author's rundown as relating more closely to Adams's early works. In addition to writing this thesis, Robinson performed and recorded *Gnarly Buttons* at the Claire Smith Performing Arts Center, University of Maryland.

179. Sanchez-Behar, Alexander. "Counterpoint and Polyphony in Recent Instrumental Works of John Adams." Ph.D. dissertation, Florida State University, 2008.

This dissertation examines Adams's works ranging from *El Dorado* (1990) to *My Father Knew Charles Ives* (2003). Since the 1990s, Adams's musical style has given greater attention to contrapuntal and polyphonic writing, as opposed to earlier works that bear more emphasis on the gradual unfoldment of harmonic regions. This study explores the melodic influences in Adams's compositions derived from Nicolas Slonimsky's *Thesaurus of Scales and Melodic Patterns*. The interaction of melodic patterns is measured using a music-theoretical similarity tool that examines the level of consonance or dissonance between two contrapuntal lines. In the realm of polyphony, the concept of dovetailing, a process of merging polyphonic textures across formal sections, is explored in Adams's orchestral works.

180. Shefcik, Matthew James. "A Performance Guide to Selected Trumpet Excerpts from the Orchestral Music of John Coolidge Adams." D.M.A. dissertation, University of Miami, 2014.

Shefick's doctoral thesis gives an overview of Adams's style of writing for the trumpet. Shefick's study examines Adams's works from 1979 onward. The works that receive greater emphasis include *Harmonielehre*, *Tromba Lontana*, *Short Ride in a Fast Machine*, *The Wound-Dresser*, *On the Transmigration of Souls*, *My Father Knew Charles Ives*, *Doctor Atomic*, and *City Noir*. Shefcik includes appendices of required mutes for each work as well as instrument ranges. Shefick documents the experiences from various renowned performers on playing Adams's works and purports that their differing perceptions of the works point to the maturation of the composer's style. Shefick aims to provide a clearer understanding of approaching Adams's trumpet parts by discussing historical, theoretical, and performance elements of Adams's works. Aspects of trumpet performance are at the forefront of Shefick's study, and to this aim, the author devotes attention to the areas concerning instrument range, endurance, technique, rhythm, intonation, and musicality.

This author asserts several works by Adams have become staples in trumpet audition lists. The works present unique challenges and innovations worthy of discussion, and previous studies or professional musicians have recognized the work's level of difficulty in trumpet literature. A few noteworthy examples include the second movement from *Harmonielehre*, which presents challenges in breath control and endurance, or *Short Ride in a Fast Machine*, which has a demanding high range and percussive articulations. After examining technical performance issues, Shefcik lists recurring threads in Adams's trumpet writing: "frequent exploitation of the upper register, the presence of long passages that test a player's endurance, rhythmic complexity, the regular requirement of extremely short articulations, wide intervallic leaps, the presence of passages that require finger dexterity and agility, the common use of swells and sudden dynamic shifts, independence of parts, and the inclusion of passages that are challenging in regards to section and ensemble playing" (78). Shefcik elaborates on these points throughout his thesis as well as in his conclusion, giving the reader a clear picture of Adams's style of writing for the trumpet.

181.   Simmons, Marc Isaac. "An Analysis of the Melodic Content of John Adams's *Harmonium*." D.M.A. dissertation, Arizona State University, 2002.

Simmons posits that while *Harmonium* is regarded as a minimalist work, its melodic content exhibits a high degree of motivic unity that owes its origin to the Western musical canon. The methodology for study entails what Simmons calls *cellular analysis*, a strategy for grouping pitch patterns into cells for comparison. The pitch patterns are measured using what Simmons refers to as normal order to represent set classes, yet his method is inconsistent, at times expressing the music-theoretical concepts of normal order and other times prime form modeled after Allen Forte. The author's biographical information of John Adams is by now outdated, and readers would benefit from consulting an updated biography, such as Sarah Cahill's entry in *Grove Music Online* (see item 303). Simmons does not include a literature review and his bibliography lacks notable publications from the 90s, including Timothy A. Johnson and Catherine Ann Pellegrino's dissertations (see items 155 and 172).

The layout of Simmons's chapters models Adams's movements: Chapter 1 is entitled "Negative Love," Chapter 2 "Because I Could Not Stop for Death," and Chapter 3 "Wild Nights!" According to Simmons, in the first movement Adams creates textural development by shifting between homophonic and polyphonic writing while maintaining crucial aspects of each cell. He explores subset relations of tetrachord and pentachord collections. Alongside the set and recurring subset relations discovered by Simmons, notions of musical form, pitch centricity, and cadential structure are discussed as they relate to the examination of each cell. One of the melodic features of the second movement entails the use of ostinati. In the analysis of "Wild Nights," Simmons examines cells with the same kinds of subset/superset relations yet finds different collections for variety and contrast to other movements. In addition to this type of cellular analysis, Simmons underscores how melodic statements either are structured in arch forms or have an ascending or descending quality. Another noteworthy aspect of *Harmonium* considers Adams's procedure for modulation where one or more vocal parts shift by a half-step motion. Adams's modulations, the author notes, normally occur at dramatic moments to facilitate structural changes within a movement.

182.   Skipp, Benjamin. "Minimalism 1960–2001: Definitions, Developments, Reception." Ph.D. dissertation, University of Oxford, 2010.

Skipp explores the development and reception of the minimalism movement from its genesis to the turn of the millennium, giving greater emphasis on more recent developments of the style, and concluding the study with Adams's *On the Transmigration of Souls*. A range of minimalist composers are included in this study: Steve Reich, Philip Glass, John Adams, Michael Nyman, John Tavener,

Louis Andriessen, and Arvo Pärt. The first chapter defines the term *minimalism* as a musical style. Skipp asserts that Adams's 2001 *On the Transmigration of Souls* does not conform to definitions of early minimalism by Timothy Johnson and other writers. According to Skipp, Adams's work contains a number of juxtapositions that prevent the motoric rhythm characteristic of earlier compositions. Furthermore, its level of dissonance and greater expressive character is foreign to the early style. Skip notes that Adams's newer style proved a formative influence on the subsequent generation of minimalists.

Skipp's second chapter considers the reception of minimalist repertoires using the Marxist concepts of humanism and structuralism. Skipp posits that the negative reception minimalism has received originates from humanist ideals embedded into formalist methods of analysis, which are ill-suited to elucidate the building blocks of minimalist works. These traditionalist music critics responded more favorably to works such as Adams's Chamber Symphony, which contains greater use of dissonance, contrast, and extra-musical references.

In the third chapter, Skipp shows how Adams and Reich transformed the early minimalist style through the integration of recorded speech and the adoption of collage techniques. Skipp notes that both composers have steered away from a pure minimalist style of writing toward more a more eclectic style. Adams's music has become synonymous with the musical expression of the present-day American experience. A noteworthy discussion in this chapter entails notions of spirituality and religion in Adams's work *On the Transmigration of Souls*.

183.   Skretta, James Edward. "Perceiving Meter in Romantic, Post-Minimal, and Electro-Pop Repertoires." D.M.A. dissertation, University of Iowa, 2015.

Skretta explores how aspects of rhythm and meter influence how listeners perceive and predict music across various styles. As a case study for minimalism, the author gives an in-depth view of Adams's *Hallelujah Junction*. Skretta's models for exploring rhythm are based on the work of numerous scholars, including but not limited to Cooper and Meyer, Lehrdahl and Jackendoff, Hasty, Krebs, Roeder, and London. Skretta's thesis seeks to elucidate confounding aural experiences where either meter is aurally divergent from its notated form, meter is not strongly asserted, or meter is ambiguous and invites multiple interpretations. The author asserts that Adams's piano work features accented patterns that thwart a listener's expectations of metric regularity. Moreover, the author strives to find some measure of objectivity on the perception of meter by assessing the dominance between two competing stimuli—a metrical accent versus a phenomenological accent, resulting from a change in volume, pitch, or duration (metrical dissonance occurs when patterns stemming from phenomenological accents conflict either one another or the notated meter signature). Skretta recomposes the opening measures from *Hallelujah Junction* to bring to light how they are ambiguous and invite different interpretations. When the second piano commences its dialogue with the first there is an abundance of metrical cues a listener must contend with; the author employs Roeder's taxonomy of accents, tracking numerous accent species such as *duration, climax,* and *nadir* to illustrate a re-notated score that corresponds with his own perception. Another rhythmic aspect Skretta explores features Kreb's notion of metrical dissonance, which is enabled by changes of texture in *Hallelujah Junction.* In creating the right conditions for metrical dissonance, Adams's rhythmic environment simultaneously interacts with formal structure, increasing in metrical dissonance or discord at texturally climactic points of the work. Overall, Skretta's engagement with scholarly sources and his analytical treatment of *Hallelujah Junction* makes this study highly relevant to the study of rhythm and meter in Adams's works as a whole.

184.   Stanton, Jason. "Thirty Years of Postminimalism: Elements and Growth." Master's thesis, California State University, Long Beach, 2010.

Stanton's thesis examines the development of the postminimalist musical style. The author considers John Adams to be one of the principal composers that shaped its development. Stanton pinpoints Adams's *China Gates* as one of the earliest postminimalist works; furthermore, he provides analytical information of the piece to compare and contrast the genesis of minimalism with Adams's musical style from this period. Stanton asserts that many aurally perceptible features in *China Gates* exhibit a departure from the earlier minimalist styles in its formal structure, harmonic motion, rhythmic complexity, and less rigid means of repetition. In his analysis of *China Gates,* Stanton charts diatonic modes employed for all formal sections, though his findings do not always coincide with other published analyses. Stanton concurs with Kyle Gann's findings, stating postminimalism introduces unpredictability and invites the composer's personal expression. Stanton also agrees with Gann's assessment of minimalism's origins as a reaction to the compositional complexities developed by serialist composers. As the postminimalist musical style developed, Stanton asserts that composers began to broaden the musical output to include multimedia works and integrated aspects of pop and rock music within the style.

185.   Stein, Joel Henry. "Volume I: Character, Symbol, and Multi-Dimensional Narrative in Three Twentieth-Century Oratorios, Volume II: *Mirror for America.*" Ph.D. dissertation, University of California, Los Angeles, 2012.

Stein's first volume investigates three twentieth-century oratorios, including Adams's *El Niño.* The author's aims are threefold: to elucidate how text and music convey characterization and narrative, to explore secondary texts and narratives that emphasize central themes from principal texts and storylines, and to illuminate how characterization and symbolism can be expressed in an oratorio. Stein remarks that storytelling in Adams's work is not linear, and the main themes are presented using seemingly unrelated narratives by both real and conceptual characters. Stein's first chapter explores elements of narrative, musical setting, action, plot, time, purpose or moral of the story, arc or layout of the oratorio, character and symbol, character interaction, and other topics. Action in *El Niño* occurs in songs where violence is expressed through a musical counterpart with loud dynamics, percussion, and short rhythmic jabs. The plot has a larger aim, focusing on salvation and the conflict of humanity to pursue a spiritual path, but there is also a more localized plot that considers the life of Joseph and Mary, and even an undercurrent of cultural conflict stemming from the multilingual text setting. The stories within Adams's oratorio manipulate time to different past events and look forward into the future. In his proper analysis, Stein delves deeper into the oratorio by examining individual arias. The author strives to give meaning to the musical foreground by connecting musical events to the text: incomplete triads suggest that salvation is incomplete, tritone relationships symbolize violence of the Great Slaughter, the high string tremolos signify the shaking of the heavens and earth, and the chorus fortissimo represents the glory of God. Although Stein's introduction gives a promising glimpse into Adams's oratorio, his analysis falls short, seldom rising above the level of word-painting considerations. This is due, in part, to a sparse bibliography that fails to incorporate necessary writings on oratorios or on Adams's earlier operas. Readers might wish to supplement Stein's analysis with more recent writings on opera and semiotics, in particular, Yayoi Uno Everett's 2015 publication *Reconfiguring Myth and Narrative in Contemporary Opera*.

186.   Strovas, Scott M. "Musical Aesthetics and Creative Identification in Two Harmonielehren by John Adams and Arnold Schoenberg." Ph.D. dissertation, Claremont Graduate University, 2012.

Strovas's musicological study explores the connection between Schoenberg's compositions, his didactic book titled *Harmonielehre*, and Adams's orchestral work bearing the same name. Strovas argues that prevalent themes from Schoenberg's work can inform analytical aspects of Adams's composition. The central thesis of Strovas's dissertation relates Schoenberg's emancipation of dissonance to Adams's unique and intuitive style of minimalism that serves as a reaction to the minimalist style itself. Thus, both composers seek to undermine the compositional development of their own time. Strovas explains that while Adams draws on minimalist devices, he integrates a dramatic element atypical of early minimalist pieces. Adams's works from the 1980s onwards reveal a more intuitive approach to composing that has been noted by K. Robert Schwarz and others; Strovas attributes this greater freedom to the composer's preliminary work on the documentary soundtrack *Matter of Heart* about the life of psychoanalyst Carl Jung. Around 1982 Adams was deeply invested in Jung's theories and underwent therapy sessions with a Jungian psychologist. Strovas traces the inception of several works by Adams as being influenced by German aesthetics, such as Jungian theory for *Harmonielehre*, Schoenberg for the Chamber Symphony, and Schiller for *Naive and Sentimental Music*.

His musical analyses reveal that although Adams employs minimalist techniques of repetition, he produces a harmonic palette more characteristic of the late Romantic era. Strovas interprets Adams's harmonic fields using tertian structures with extended notes in a manner that parallels analysis of jazz harmony—this approach diverges from Timothy A. Johnson's analytical tools on understanding

Adams's harmonies. Strovas's approach of employing stratification to entire fields of sound is markedly different from Johnson's theoretical model for analysis. In Strovas's examination of *Harmonielehre*, the author highlights the technique of stratified layers; namely, the independence of melody above motoric pulsations and brass entrances. This issue touches upon Adams's intuitive postminimalist style; Strovas draws a parallel to jazz in Adams's improvisatory style. Moreover, this idea coincides with later works where the orchestra maintains homophonic textures, such as in the first movement of his Violin Concerto. Contributing to its improvisatory nature, Strovas concurs with Johnson and Pellegrino that Adams's music often unfolds in unpredictable ways, thus distancing its stylistic signature from early minimalist techniques. Later on, Strovas attempts to describe formal aspects of *Harmonielehre* bearing in mind thematic considerations, referring to themes by number, and characterizing them as minimalist, Romantic, or lyrical.

The second portion of Strovas's dissertation addresses a host of other topics, including Adams's works *Light Over Water* and *On the Transmigration of Souls*, and Adams's thoughts on Schoenberg and his pupil Leon Kirchner, who later became Adams's teacher. The connection between Schoenberg's *Farben* and Adams's *Harmonielehre*, relating textures, orchestration, and arrangement of dynamics, is given treatment in Strovas's discussions along with musical examples in this portion. Strovas's dissertation, together with Derfler's 1998 study on Adams and Schoenberg (see item 140), provides readers with an in-depth perspective of *Harmonielehre* through a contextualization of the work and close analysis.

187. Taylor, Anthony Gordon. "John Adams's "Gnarly Buttons": Issues of History, Performance, and Style." D.M.A. dissertation, University of Cincinnati, 2007.

Taylor remarks that *Gnarly Buttons* has not received enough attention in scholarly writings. The author's intent in writing his dissertation is to affirm the importance of this clarinet concerto in respect to the composer's oeuvre. Taylor traces the history of the concerto, organizing this study into five sections: *Gnarly Buttons* in context; the birth of *Gnarly Buttons*; a performance guide; Adams, the first generation of minimalists, and Stravinsky; and compositional and stylistic analysis of *Gnarly Buttons*.

In the first chapter, Taylor gives a general rundown of the individual movements of the concerto. He notes that in the first movement, the scoring of the opening measures originally contained a doubled synthesizer part along with the clarinet. For the second movement, Taylor posits it combines Stravinsky's neo-classical style from *L'Histoire du soldat* and *Three Pieces* with vernacular American jazz and bluegrass. Taylor references Adams, who states that the third movement of the concerto expands upon the harmonic language from the "Chorus of Exiled Palestinians" from *The Death of Klinghoffer*. In his second chapter, Taylor devotes attention to the critical reception of the work, among other things, noting it had received favorable reviews. Taylor also provides readers with a discography for the concerto. Following Taylor's attendance of a rehearsal with the Los Angeles

Philharmonic, led by Adams, Taylor interviews accomplished performers on rehearsal and performance aspects of the work—this is presented in the third chapter. Detailed practice tips targeting difficult passages are discussed along with related performance issues, such as coordinating the solo clarinet part with the orchestra. Timing issues are also at the forefront of Taylor's discussion, taking into account the conductor's role in keeping time. Taylor advocates analysis of the individual movements for a more informed performance. For instance, in the third movement, Taylor confirms Adams's assertion that the onomato-poeic motive "Put Your Loving Arms Around Me" is directly webbed to chord changes. In the fourth chapter, Taylor finds common traits in Adams's musical style to that of first-generation minimalists. According to the author, Adams's use of harmonic progression is influenced by Reich's own style—Taylor illustrates this point using excerpts from *The Chairman Dances* and *Lollapalooza*. The next portion of this chapter discusses the connection between Adams's two fanfares for orchestra (*Tromba Lontata* and *Short Ride in a Fast Machine*) as being influ-enced by Stravinsky's ballet *Petrushka*. The last section of the dissertation focuses on analytical aspects of the concerto, tracing earlier minimalist elements from *Nixon in China* as well as its more recent compositional traits from *The Death of Klinghoffer*. Taylor presents an adapted form of Timothy A. Johnson's formalized method of analysis designed specifically for the music of Adams.

For the purposes of this study, Taylor conducted interviews with Adams; Michael Collins, who premiered the work; Paul Meecham; William Helmers, clarinetist soloist who performed the North American premiere; Sean Osborn, former clar-inetist of the Metropolitan Opera Orchestra; and several other accomplished musicians who had collaborated with Adams on *Gnarly Buttons* in some capac-ity. The interview with Michael Collins touches on performance issues primar-ily, and Collins's thoughts on whether Adams's concerto feels idiomatic for the solo instrument. In the interview with Sean Osborn, he discusses the individual movements at length and provides insight into the title of the work as a tribute to Adams's father and his struggles with Alzheimer's disease—the third movement is most directly influenced by his father's condition. Osborn states that the first movement of the concerto makes clear references to Carl Nielsen's Clarinet Con-certo, op. 57. Of the three movements from *Gnarly Buttons*, Osborn believes the first is the most technical and hardest to memorize. In speaking with Paul Mee-cham, the title of the second movement, "Hoedown (Mad Cow)," is explained as influenced by the mad cow disease scare at the time of composition. In the interview with John Adams, the author and composer discuss the folk-like nature of the first movement as being subconsciously influenced by Stravinsky's *Three Pieces*. Adams contextualizes the concerto vis-à-vis earlier works to show a departure from his earlier minimalist style. Adams, who is at times critical of his own works, expresses his satisfaction for *Gnarly Buttons*, notably, for its develop-ment of a unique harmonic style. Adams references *Naive and Sentimental Music* for its similar treatment of the harmonic parameter as its germinating idea for the composition.

188.   Tedford, David. "Performing the Canon or Creating Inroads: A Study of Higher Education Orchestral Programming of Contemporary Music." D.M.A. dissertation, University of Iowa, 2015.

Tedford's study examines college conductors' contemporary repertoire from 1990 onwards, including Adams's *On the Transmigration of Souls* and *City Noir*. The author contemplates the importance and appeal of contemporary music for conductors. Tedford's information is derived out of a written survey administered to 297 higher education orchestra conductors—the survey questions are included in his study. The author gives a breakdown of contemporary-music performances across college symphony orchestras and bands, professional orchestras, and youth symphonies. John Adams receives a top rank for the highest number of performances by professional orchestras, though not for collegiate orchestras. Tedford asserts that the level of difficulty of Adams's works may be a contributing factor for fewer collegiate performances. Adams's instrumentation may prove to be another complication, as most of his works contain keyboard samplers and requirements for specific software. In recent years, Adams has simplified this challenge by entrusting Mark Grey with technical support issues pertaining to his works. Grey has developed a website that outlines all technical information for programing Adams's works, accessible at https://mhgrey.wordpress.com.

189.   Teichler, Robert Christopher. "An Analysis of John Adams's *Lollapalooza*." D.M.A. dissertation, Northwestern University, 2006.

Teichler provides an analysis of Adams's *Lollapalooza*, beginning his study with some general statements regarding its tripartite structure and its eclectic postminimalist style infused with vestiges of pop music and jazz. The author comments on Adams's notated triple meter without elaborating on conflicting aurally perceived meters; thus, readers might consult other scholarly studies to gain an understanding of rhythm and meter in Adams's works (see items 52, 183, and 274). Teichler suggests that formal sections are delineated by aspects of instrumental range and orchestration. He touches upon some notable features of the music, such as thematic ideas and their association to tonal centers. Teichler notes thematic sections are predominantly diatonic, while chromaticism is reserved strictly for a prominent transitional passage near the middle of the work. The author catalogs prominent motivic patterns from Adams's *Lollapalooza* numerically and chronologically (in order of entry) in his first appendix. Indeed, the strongest point of Teichler's study lies in his catalog of motivic elements and their development throughout Adams's musical work. As a minor quibble, Teichler does not cite Adams in regards to the onomatopoetic qualities of *Lollapalooza* as they relate to the thematic aspects of the work. Another shortcoming of Teichler's analysis is his analytical presentation, which begs for a more coherent organization and structured method stemming from pertinent writings on pitch centricity, musical layering, and other subjects explored in this study.

190.   Thompson, Brian. "*Nixon in China*: Grand Opera and the 'Avant-Garde.'" Master's thesis, University of Victoria, 1991.

Thompson's study frames Adams's *Nixon in China* within twentieth-century opera and American culture. The author assesses its dramatic nature and level of success. Chapter 1 examines Adams's libretto and the staging of the world premiere with the Houston Grand Opera. Thompson begins with a first-rate synopsis of the opera, relating the opera characters, acting, and musical aspects to the principal plot line. Thompson gives an in-depth look at Goodman's libretto, reflecting on gender and cultural differences between opposing characters.

Chapter 2 introduces signature traits of Adams's musical language, encompassing compositional procedures, Adams's use of texture, and musical form. Like numerous other writers, Thompson pegs Adams as a romantic minimalist. The defining characteristics of Adams's style are constant pulse, repetition, ostinatos, and arpeggios. In the area of rhythm and meter, Thompson brands Adams's writing as straightforward, using quarter notes and eighth notes predominantly and metric modulations with less frequency. The author holds the same viewpoint toward Adams's harmonies, stating that the composer molds triads and seventh chords in a clear manner. Thompson pinpoints two types of modulation along with their dramatic effect in the realm of opera writing. Other compositional techniques are discussed, including the use of alternating harmonies, instrumentation, the dramatic effect of contrasting material, melody and text-setting qualities given to each of the characters, and form reflected more closely to operatic tradition than minimalist structures. Thompson correlates text and action throughout the entire opera to the concurrent musical textures composed by Adams. According to Thompson, Adams's integration of diverse materials, historical references, and ironic quotations all serve to distance their style from early minimalism.

In Chapter 3, Thompson addresses the premiere's critical reception. The author notes that most reviewers viewed the libretto favorably yet had qualms about the politics that propel the opera, Adams's musical style, or the staging. Thompson notes that some of the harshest reviews came from opera specialists rather than music critics.

The fourth and final chapter, subtitled "The Return to Grand Opera," explores main historical trends in twentieth-century opera tradition as a means for contextualization and critical assessment of Adams's opera. The trend in opera during this time was reflected by smaller-scale chamber operas that contained an introspective subject matter. After the Second World War, experimental composers generally avoided writing opera music. In some respects, Thompson asserts that *Nixon in China* represents a conservative, postmodern approach to opera writing; namely, the return to subjectivity and romanticism and the sense of grand opera associated with nineteenth-century opera composers. The author's own review of this operatic work is that characters are mythologized and their negotiations are downplayed, which obscures the creators' stance on the subject and detracts from the coherence of the opera. As a minor quibble to an otherwise informative thesis, Thompson's musical examples could be illustrated more effectively with titles and score annotations to illustrate his points.

191. Traficante, Debra Lee. "An Analysis of John Adams' *Grand Pianola Music*." D.M.A. dissertation, University of Oklahoma, 2010.

Traficante's doctoral thesis provides an in-depth examination of *Grand Pianola Music*. This is a work that Adams regards highly, yet it has received harsh criticism for its boisterous statement against avant-garde composers and satire of the classical style. Traficante acquaints readers with background information of the work derived from Adams's own writings. Adams had a dream of driving on Interstate 5. He observed two limousines approached him, and as they passed they morphed into Steinway grand pianos playing B-flat and E-flat major arpeggios. Traficante includes information of the premiere, subsequent performances, and available recordings. Following prefatory information of *Grand Pianola Music*, Traficante devotes attention to analytical issues such as scoring, instrumentation, an exploration of key areas, and analysis of its formal structure. The author's analysis of key areas does not formalize any preference rules for segmentation in Adams's work nor outline prerequisites for establishing pitch centers, and thus gives the impression of makeshift approach that cannot be readily duplicated for other musical works. Traficante asserts the importance of the golden ratio in Adams's work, and to this aim, she offers illustrations that chart dynamic levels and their connection between the final apex and the golden ratio. The concluding portion of Traficante's study is geared toward conductors such as herself. The author offers an insider's perspective for conducting this work, along with tips on rehearsing and performing, and in particular, highlighting the final peak in close proximity to the golden ratio.

192. Vazquez-Ramos, Angel M. "Maria Guinand: Conductor, Teacher, and Promoter of Latin American Choral Music." Ph.D. dissertation, Florida State University, 2010.

Vazquez-Ramos describes Maria Guinand's role of Choir Master of the *Schola Cantorum de Venezuela* in John Adams's 2006 world premiere of *A Flowering Tree*. She also receives credit as Choir Master and Artistic Director for the 2008 Nonesuch 327100-2 recording of this opera, together with the London Symphony Orchestra, under the baton of Maestro Adams. Although Vazquez-Ramos's dissertation is published in English, the author includes an interview with Guinand in Spanish, where the internationally renowned choral conductor recounts meeting Adams as well as their collaboration of the opera.

193. Wyman, Richard E. "A Wind Ensemble Transcription of Part 1 (the First Movement) of *Harmonielehre* by John Adams with Commentary." D.M.A. dissertation, University of Connecticut, 2014.

Wyman's dissertation demonstrates his process of transcribing the first movement of *Harmonielehre* for wind ensemble. His commentary includes two chapters devoted to the historical and theoretical context of minimalism and the music of John Adams. The final chapter describes in detail his methodology for transcribing the work. Wyman details how instrument families are treated in his transcription, giving each their unique function and narrative. Wyman lists other works by Adams that have also been transcribed for wind ensemble: *Lollapalooza*, transcribed by John Spinazzola; *Short Ride in a Fast Machine*, transcribed by Lawrence Gordon; and *The Chairman Dances*, transcribed by Cormac Cannon.

194.   Zorgniotti, Marc F. "Quotations and Constructivism in Twentieth-Century Violin Chaconnes by John Adams, Hans W. Henze, and Moses Pergament." D.M.A. dissertation, University of Cincinnati, 2010.

Zorgniotti examines three violin *chaconnes* from the twentieth century, including Adams's chaconne from the second movement of his 1993 Violin Concerto, titled "Body through Which the Dream Flows" after a poem by Robert Hass. The author describes how Adams's chaconne stems from continuous-variation practice closely associated with ostinato genres. Moreover, Adams's musical borrowing, in the form of direct quotations, alludes to Baroque composers; specifically, Pachelbel's celebrated *Canon in D*. Zorgniotti references Rebecca Jemian and Anne Marie de Zeeuw's 1996 interview with Adams (see item 101), which touches on many of the same issues in the Violin Concerto. Zorgniotti's introduction traces the origins of the Chaconne and finds a working definition for his study. According to the author, a chaconne bears the following recurring characteristics: (1) a repeating harmonic or melodic pattern often supported by an ostinato, (2) a formal organization of continuous variation, (3) a predominant use of the minor mode, and (4) a solemn affect. The author traces the origins of the genre and discusses its standard phrase opening using the harmonic progression tonic-dominant-submediant, which Adams models after Pachelbel's Canon. Zorgniotti believes that Adams's Chaconne shows two prominent aspects of Adams's compositional style, the first being a dialogue with composers of the past and the second being a preoccupation for gradual processes. Zorgniotti notes that twenty-one out of twenty-nine total iterations from Pachelbel's bass ostinato appear in the original key. Adams gradually modernizes the canon, saturating passages with tritones, transforming the rhythm through diminution and augmentation, and overlapping and displacing notes. Further modernization is achieved through electronic music, minimalist passages, a preponderance of percussion instruments, and the use of quarter-tone intonations. Zorgniotti maps the formal design of Adams's movement to elucidate bass ostinato statements, tonal centers, and main features that delineate each section. The author includes score images of Adams's quarter-tone technique, polyrhythms, and minimalist-style passages, yet the low picture quality renders them unusable—readers can view the score online through Adams's publisher, Boosey & Hawkes. Overall, Zorgniotti raises interesting points, though many have already been iterated in a previous interview with the composer. A discussion of the melodic elements from Adams's chaconne can also be found in my 2015 *Music Theory Spectrum* article.

7

Select Newspaper Titles, News Articles, and Reviews

195.   *Chicago Tribune.* www.chicagotribune.com.

   The *Chicago Tribune* contains a great number of articles on Adams. Many articles are written by *Chicago Tribune* music critic John von Rhein and published from the mid-1980s to present time. These newspaper articles provide much more than performance critiques—though critiques form an essential part of any newspaper column. Articles contain information about the composer's views on myriad subjects, interviews with Adams, and other material germane to the study of his works. Various noteworthy articles discuss topics ranging from compositional development, collaboration with the *Lyric Opera of Chicago*, the composer's religious views and their influence on *El Niño* and other works, composition achievements and awards, the composer's act of balancing the yin (composition) and yang (conducting), and thoughts on Adams's synthesis of musical styles.

196.   *The Guardian.* www.theguardian.com/us.

   The British newspaper *The Guardian* contains a wide variety of articles on Adams and his musical works. Many of these articles are written by Fiona Maddocks, who is the chief music critic for the newspaper. Other frequent contributors appear, including Andrew Clements and Tom Service. The online version of the newspaper contains a few articles that introduce Adams's music and the style of minimalism, such as "A Guide to John Adams's Music." Recording reviews make up a portion of their music articles, including reviews of Adams's *Grand Pianola Music*, the Violin Concerto, *My Father Knew Charles Ives*, *The Dharma at Big Sur*, *Absolute Jest*, and the Berliner Philharmoniker 4-CD recordings from 2017.

Performance reviews of several recent compositions also appear in print for *Doctor Atomic*, *Scheherazade.2*, and *Guide to Strange Places*. Other articles delve into relevant subjects about Adams's orchestral and operatic works, including but not limited to the following: Adams's views on politics and the political overlap in *Nixon in China*, the composer's indifference for Pierre Boulez's musical aesthetic, the *Klinghoffer* controversy, the making of *Doctor Atomic*, a lengthy interview with librettist Alice Goodman on collaborating with Adams, the *Metropolitan Opera* cancellation of *The Death of Klinghoffer* simulcast, and thoughts on composing *A Flowering Tree*. Additionally, there are interviews with Adams himself, who discusses a wide range of topics about his works, his views on the state of classical music, and his ongoing composition projects. Several of these publications are accompanied by audio excerpts from his musical works as well as recorded interviews.

197. *Los Angeles Times*. www.latimes.com.

For decades, Adams has influenced classical circles in Los Angeles through premieres of his works, some of which are dedicated to important musical figures in the Los Angeles area, such as Esa Pekka Salonen and Gustavo Dudamel. Adams is also showcased as a perennial guest conductor for the Los Angeles Philharmonic. A great number of music articles on Adams are written by classical music critic Mark Swed. While the articles tend to be concise in length, they include important statements by Adams that encapsulate larger themes in his music and other thoughts often missing in lengthier interviews. In one such example from a 2012 article with Reed Johnson, Adams admits to having a period of spiritual self-doubt while working on the subject of *The Gospel According to the Other Mary*. While self-doubt for an art form as introspective as music can be healthy for a composer, and certainly Adams has experienced these periods, such as his compositional crisis following *Nixon in China*, this begs the question of whether (and how) spiritual doubt is reflected in the characters, the subject matter, and the music from his recent opera.

198. *The New York Times*. www.nytimes.com.

The New York Times is one of the most important news publications containing a wealth of material on Adams. Some noteworthy pieces include information and critical reviews of his earlier operas, including Richard Taruskin's 2001 article that heightened the *Klinghoffer* controversy. In addition to premiere critiques, the newspaper provides performance announcements, recording reviews, and information on commissions and awards. The content in most of these publications should not be regarded as superficial; they contain Adams's thoughts on his works, his mode of composition, and inspirational sources. John Rockwell's September 17, 2002 article on the commission for *On the Transmigration of Souls* highlights facets of Adams's intuitive compositional approach, detailing his use of technology and thoughts on his artistic aim for the work. In an informative review of Adams's *Gospel* dated April 2, 2017, Zachary Woolfe asserts that Adams has not received enough credit as a lyrical composer, citing a number of examples from Adams's oeuvre that show evidence of his lyrical writing. Adams himself published a *New York Times* review of Stephen Walsh's 2018 book titled *Debussy: A Painter in Sound* on November 19, 2018. Though Adams doesn't attribute his musical influences to Debussy and the impressionist school, he shows interest in his music as evidenced by his own orchestral arrangement of Debussy's *Cinq poèmes de Charles Baudelaire* titled *Le Livre de Baudelaire*. Adams regards Debussy as a composer who liberated harmony, producing, when combined with his use of whole-tone scales, music that "felt exceptionally free of the angst and highly charged emotionalism of most of the Romantic repertoire." I suspect Adams sought to expand his orchestrational craftsmanship, and Debussy's works lend themselves well to this fruitful exercise. Additionally, the connection between Debussy and Adams is underplayed in scholarly studies, to date. Adams's undulating dominant-seventh chords in *Nixon in China* bear an uncanny resemblance to Debussy's free-flowing and impressionist harmonic treatment.

199.   *San Francisco Chronicle.* www.sfchronicle.com.

The *San Francisco Chronicle* contains news on Adams's upcoming concerts, recording and performance reviews, and other articles geared to familiarize readers with their local composer. The in-house music critic Joshua Kosman is the most frequent contributor of these news pieces. Kosman is a longtime proponent of Adams's music, which he considers expressive, multifaceted, and having an eclectic style, which has found common ground in Mozart, Ravel, Glass, and even personalities such as Frank Zappa. Noteworthy articles from this newspaper delve deeper than basic descriptions of Adams's works and style of composition. For instance, in the November 1, 1992 article on Adams's *Klinghoffer*, music critic Robert Commanday announces the premiere of the San Francisco production of this opera. If his words are any sign of the opera's longevity, the city of San Francisco seems ready to embrace Adams's opera despite its controversies resulting from other productions. In Kosman's April 8, 2003 piece honoring Adams for his recent Pulitzer Prize, the composer is candid about his views on the Pulitzer Board's history of awarding composers deemed stylistically academic and conservative. Kosman's December 3, 2007 article brings to light unique facets of Adams's compositional development, asserting that Adams's *Son of Chamber Symphony* creates a single overarching narrative enabled by a newfound symphonic approach to writing chamber music. In the January 19, 2015 music column, Kosman writes a short study detailing Adams's fascination for Beethoven's music, as exemplified by *Grand Pianola Music*, *Absolute Jest*, and his second string quartet.

SINGLE-AUTHORED ARTICLES AND REVIEWS

200.   Allen, David. "Conducting an Eerie, Political 'Gospel.'" *The New York Times* (March 26, 2017). www.nytimes.com/2017/03/26/arts/music/david-robertson-john-adams.html?ref=topics.

Allen interviews David Robertson, who is the music director of the St. Louis Symphony and has released multiple recordings of Adams's works. The two discuss Adams's recent oratorio *The Gospel According to the Other Mary*, in preparation for the March 31, 2017 Carnegie Hall performance under the baton of Maestro Robertson. Allen notes that the oratorio has been revised extensively since its world premiere in 2012. According to Allen, *Gospel* conflates the story of Jesus's death with recent themes of social justice. Robertson describes Adams's musical aesthetic as a dramatic one, albeit from the lens of minimalist techniques. Over the years, Adams has expanded dramatic musical structures from smaller works to larger operatic and theatrical works. Notions of spirituality and politics are intertwined in the oratorio, which Allen explains as a result of the composer's longtime collaboration with Peter Sellars. Adams's musical lines for the countertenors remind Robertson of Mozart's *Die Zauberflöte*, and the conductor ponders whether Adams deliberately hearkened back to the spirit of Mozart. Robertson explains Adams's harmonic structures as a combination of dissonant harmonies with old-sounding consonant harmonies reserved for special moments. Adams's orchestration of these harmonies creates colors and textures in a manner that depicts an evolving process. While Robertson's concise description of the oratorio paints a general introduction to the work, I would have also expected him to discuss rehearsal and performance issues that pertain to Adams's *Gospel*.

201. Barone, Joshua. "Adès and Adams: Big Composers with Simultaneous Big Premieres." *The New York Times* (March 6, 2019). www.nytimes.com/2019/03/06/arts/music/john-adams-thomas-ades-piano.html.

Barone writes about the upcoming world premiere of Adams's latest piano concerto titled *Must the Devil Have All the Good Tunes?* The author's description of the work and other relevant information stems from, in part, Adams's Official Website (www.earbox.com). Adams's own conception of his latest piano concerto admittedly conjures Liszt's *Totentanz*, though painted with an American signature.

202. Bernheimer, Martin. "OPERA REVIEW: Sellars, et al, on the Fault Line: New Song-Play Barely Registers on Richter Scale." *Los Angeles Times* (May 15, 1995). www.latimes.com/archives/la-xpm-1995-05-15-ca-952-story.html.

Following the world premiere of *I Was Looking at the Ceiling and Then I Saw the Sky* in May 1995, the *Los Angeles Times* music critic Martin Bernheimer wrote a scathing review of Adams's songplay, referring to the work as "a mess." For starters, Bernheimer claimed that the singers were unimpressive and their walking on stage, singing into hand-held microphones, proved to be clumsy—subsequent performances changed this aspect, opting for body microphones. This critic contends that the songplay's visual elements—two mural drops that depict Los Angeles and vinyl banners created by a consortium of graffiti artists—far outweighed the music, libretto, and staging in terms of quality. Bernheimer scorns this collaboration for nearly every aspect one can imagine: the acts supposedly go on forever, the collage of musical styles hides Adams's own voice, and this author even asks whether the two spoken poems are a result of an incomplete creation. Sellars is not immune to the harsh criticism of Bernheimer, who states that Sellars allows the characters to "strike poster poses" and "stand around on an empty stage." For a contrasting review, readers may wish to examine Mark Swed's 2014 article, also published in the *Los Angeles Times*.

203.   Cahill, Sarah. "I Was Looking at the Ceiling and Then I Saw the Sky." *East Bay Express* (May 19, 1995). Reprinted in *The John Adams Reader: Essential Writings on an American Composer*, ed. Thomas May, 345–9. Pompton Plains: Amadeus, 2006.

Just a week following the premiere of Adams's *I Was Looking at the Ceiling and Then I Saw the Sky*, Cahill gives her impressions of the work. As Cahill notes, the work is difficult to categorize as either an opera, a musical, or a new kind of genre altogether. But Adams's "songplay" has not received the attention that Cahill predicted it would, believing it would have greater success because of its crossover between opera and musical theater. It seems that at present time neither opera lovers nor musical theater enthusiasts have adopted the work into their fold. The songplay's synopsis deals with the 1994 Northridge earthquake and the impact the disaster had on the lives of seven young characters. Looking into their lives, Adams and librettist June Jordan delve into difficult topics such as immigration, birth control, and racism. Jordan's colloquial style of writing is a polar opposite of Adams's first librettist, Alice Goodman, who favors highly stylized, rhymed pentameter in her prose. But Jordan's language seems more natural to the lives of these seven characters who share the challenges of living in a neighborhood of the Los Angeles metropolis. Cahill praises Adams's musical setting of the libretto, stating "it's as if Adams took Jordan's text and spoke it over and over until he found the natural cadences and melodic contours of each phrase, and then composed the music to fit"—her remark is likely not far from the truth (347). Cahill observes that parts of the songplay are self-referential: one of the character's solos, titled "Donde Estas?" reminisces Adams's 1993 album *Hoodoo Zephyr*. There are also echoes from *Christian Zeal and Activity*, and even from *Klinghoffer*. Cahill speaks of the eclectic nature of the songplay, including songs in different styles, such as pop, jazz, gospel, blues, funk, minimalism, and others. The result is laudable, though I suspect audiences and critics may have not been able to reconcile such musical variety within a single artistic work. The work belongs to its own category, Cahill confirms.

204.   Cooper, Michael. "John Adams Writes a New Opera, and It's a Western." *The New York Times* (November 16, 2017). www.nytimes.com/2017/11/16/arts/music/john-adams-opera-san-francisco-girls.html?smid=pl-share.

Cooper interviews Adams two days before the composer's world premiere of his latest opera, *Girls of the Golden West*. Beneath the surface of the opera's gold rush storyline lie unfiltered events containing ethnic tensions and brutality towards women. The libretto has been compiled by Sellars and Adams from Mark Twain,

Shakespeare (miners enjoyed his plays), and Louise Knapp Smith Clappe's *Dame Shirley* letters. Adams relays to Cooper that many people came to California looking for gold, "and when it became not so easy to find gold, they all started sounding like Donald Trump." Adams amusingly discusses this contemporary parallel, and yet over the years he has strongly opposed the nickname of "political" composer. Adams elaborates on one of the opera's characters named Josefa Segovia, based on a real Mexican immigrant who was lynched by an angry mob for killing a white miner in self-defense. Adams recalls writing choruses for the angry mob during the 2016 presidential debate when the news showed footage of Donald Trump supporters yelling "lock her up!" in reference to Hillary Clinton.

Adams speaks of his uncertainty about the seemingly diminishing effect composers bear on contemporary society, a frustration he has voiced in other interviews as well, particularly in regards to classical music not being able to break into popular culture today. Some of the more memorable moments from this opera include an aria based on Frederick Douglass's "What to the Slave is the Fourth of July," the instrumental interlude for Lola Montez's "Spider Dance," and original music based on miners' songs from the gold rush period. Adams speaks briefly about his sparse textures and lucid harmonies being more fitting than a modernist, complex harmonic language. Adams predicts that *Girls of the Golden West* will be his last large-scale opera, and he will prefer to engage in smaller projects in the future.

205.   Dicker, Matthew. "Composer John Adams Making Old Musical Forms New." *The Washington Times* (May 17, 2013). www.washingtontimes.com/news/2013/may/17/not-the-same-old-music/.

This article announces Adams's 2012–2013 residency in the Library of Congress and also provides portions of an interview with the composer. Dicker aims to persuade readers that contemporary classical music is relevant in today's world. The author underlines serious subjects—terrorism, war, greed and power in politics—from John Adams's operas that have impacted modern society in significant ways. During his residency, Adams is tasked with upcoming concerts and handpicking a musical work for commission from another composer. Following these concerts, the U.S. Army Blues presents a big-band concert, showcasing the kind of music familiar to Adams from his days as a youth spent at the Winnipesaukee Gardens. Adams considers big-band music America's indigenous sound and regrets that few people enjoy listening. The composer also states that his own style of writing for orchestra is heavily influenced by Ellington, Count Basie, and Benny Goodman's band.

206.   Davidson, Justin. "History's Unholy Trinity (*Doctor Atomic*)." *Newsday* (October 3, 2005). Reprinted in *The John Adams Reader: Essential Writings on an American Composer*, ed. Thomas May, 379–81. Pompton Plains: Amadeus, 2006.

Davidson published his review of *Doctor Atomic* two days following its world premiere, performed with the San Francisco Opera. The author articulates Adams's biggest achievement in this opera is the absorption of compressed anxieties from the World War II era into the "music's own flesh" (379). This is accomplished through a slew of extra-musical sounds, including alarms, screams, metallic grindings, and tunes that peer through radio static. Musically, the orchestra aids in the feeling of anxiety through timpani rumbles and staccato chords played by the strings. According to Davidson, Adams's countdown of the atomic bomb is treated through changes in tempo, tone, short horn blasts, percussive strings, and tremolo. This interpretation of the countdown has been the subject of Yayoi Uno Everett's 2012 study from the standpoint of music semiotics. Davidson asserts that Adams's style of writing in this opera shows the same qualities as his earlier works. One of the most memorable arias of the opera incorporates John Donne's poem "Batter My Heart, Three-Person'd God"; Davidson finds the aria reminiscent of John Dowland's music. Not much is stated of the other characters in the opera, aside from the fact that the other men are figures of doubt, while Kitty Oppenheimer embodies much of the soul of the opera.

207.   Dyer, Richard. "Adams, Sellars Think Smaller in New Opera (*I Was Looking at the Ceiling and Then I Saw the Sky*)." *The Boston Globe* (July 23, 1995). Reprinted in *The John Adams Reader: Essential Writings on an American Composer*, ed. Thomas May, 350–4. Pompton Plains: Amadeus, 2006.

Dyer opines that Adams's "songplay" *I Was Looking at the Ceiling and Then I Saw the Sky* attempts to tackle important themes, yet the result falls short of expectations. Dyer believes that Adams's work has assimilated small-scale operas by Britten and Brecht/Weill as well as *Porgy and Bess*, *West Side Story*, and pop albums such as *Abbey Road*, *Tommy*, and *John Wesley Harding*. The author asserts that the subtext of the work explores the impact of societal walls on the individual lives of the characters. He defines Jordan's writing as having a sophisticated sense of urban rhythm, yet lacking the ability to create compellingly complex characters or convincing dramatic events. For Dyer, the characters are clichés because they are not believable. This critic speaks with a general approval of Adams's scoring and remarks that even a few of the songs have breakthrough potential. In fact, Dyer believes Adams's songplay is more successful than his earlier operas. In contradiction, Dyer purports that his music lacks in shading, depth, complexity, and expression of the characters.

208.   Gelt, Jessica. "'Available Light,' A Performance Art Landmark, Makes the Leap from 1983 to 2015." *Los Angeles Times* (June 4, 2015). www.latimes.com/entertain ment/arts/la-et-cm-available-light-childs-adams-gehry-20150604-story.html.

Gelt remarks that *Available Light* has gained renewed interest in recent years. Following its return premiere at the Walt Disney Concert Hall on June 5, 2015, the work will be showcased on tour internationally. Gelt looks into aspects of the performance work from its three collaborators: Childs's choreography, Gehry's staging, and Adams's music. Adams claims to have made several additions to his score to give dancers a greater sense of pulsation and facilitate the merging of music and dance. Gelt touches on the development of Adams's score, originating as a multichannel electronic work, subsequently adding brass instruments for the studio recording in San Francisco, and now undergoing further updates.

209.   Ginell, Richard S. "John Adams Delivers a Devil of a New Concerto. Yuja Wang Pounds It Out." *Los Angeles Times* (March 8, 2019). www.latimes.com/entertain ment/arts/la-et-cm-john-adams-devil-review-20190308-story.html.

Ginell expresses Adams has a penchant for catchy titles, as is the case with his third piano concerto, *Must the Devil Have All the Good Tunes?*, premiered on March 7, 2019. In addition to the piano part composed specifically for pianist Yuja Wang, Ginell indicates there is a honky-tonk synthesizer part, though its sound was masked by the entire ensemble. This critic states there are only few memorable themes in Adams's work, the most notable stemming from a quotation of Henry Mancini's *Peter Gunn*.

210.   Henahan, Donal. "Opera: 'Nixon in China.'" *The New York Times* (October 24, 1987). www.nytimes.com/1987/10/24/arts/opera-nixon-in-china.html.

Music critic for the *New York Times* and winner of the Pulitzer Prize for Criticism Donal Henahan writes a scathing review of the *Nixon in China* premiere. Henahan wrote one of the most famous (and humorous) attacks of Adams's music: "Mr. Adams does for the arpeggio what McDonald's did for the hamburger, grinding out one simple idea unto eternity." According to Henahan, the libretto is a "good-natured skit, but not the political or social satire one might expect." Henahan opines the main problem stems from the music, describing it as mechanical and uneventful. Perhaps this critic's most disparaging remark is that *Nixon in China* is hardly a strong candidate for standard repertoire.

211.   Kisselgoff, Anna. "BALLET REVIEW: What's Black and White and Rhythmic All Over? Ask Peter Martins." *The New York Times* (January 24, 2002). www.nytimes. com/2002/01/24/arts/ballet-review-what-s-black-and-white-and-rhythmic-all-over-ask-peter-martins.html.

Kisselgoff details how choreographer of the *New York City Ballet* Peter Martins set his most recent ballet to Adams's *Hallelujah Junction*. Peter Martins presented the world premiere of his choreography on March 24, 2001, with the Royal Danish Theatre in Copenhagen; the New York City Ballet premiere took place on January 22, 2002. Kisselgoff elaborates on issues of lighting, the staging of the pianists and dancers, and dancers' attire. In the remainder of the review, Kisselgoff describes the manner in which the ballet dancers depict Adams's music in each of the movements.

212.   Kosman, Joshua. "Symphony Premieres Adams's Splendid *Ives*." *San Francisco Chronicle* (May 2, 2003). Reprinted in *The John Adams Reader: Essential Writings on an American Composer*, ed. Thomas May, 376–8. Pompton Plains: Amadeus, 2006.

Kosman reviews Adams's orchestral work *My Father Knew Charles Ives* shortly after its world premiere with the *San Francisco Symphony*. Like other music critics, Kosman hopes to impart a memorable description of the work under discussion, and as such, his comments reveal a penchant for hyperbole. The author claims the emotional experiences of earlier works are nothing compared to those of Adams's *Ives*. Kosman perceives Adams's symphony as a funny, rueful, and heartbreaking musical memoir. He hails Adams's *Ives* as a work that charts new directions for the composer's rhythmic language and his use of the orchestra, though the author does not provide more detail on how Adams forges a new creative period. Kosman asserts that the first movement of the work, titled "Concord," is suggestive of Ives's Piano Sonata No. 2, which bears the same name. The first movement is one of pastiche: listeners sojourn to the world of marches and hymn tunes, colliding with other musical fragments, including a reveille and a Beethoven duet that Adams played as a budding clarinet student. The second movement, titled "The Lake," recreates the dance hall where Adams's parents met. Adams's orchestration opens with "shimmering, slow-moving string harmonies punctuated by blurry twitterings from the woodwinds and percussion, like sonic fireflies on a long-ago summer evening"—I wonder whether this is what Kosman perceives as forging a new orchestral path (377). According to Kosman, the last movement, titled "The Mountain," is less unified. The premiere performance is relayed as lackluster, yet it does not permanently blemish the strength of this new addition to symphonic repertoire.

213. ____. "Voice of America: Composer John Adams Speaks for the Nation." *San Francisco Chronicle* (May 18, 2003). Reprinted in *The John Adams Reader: Essential Writings on an American Composer*, ed. Thomas May, 59–62. Pompton Plains: Amadeus, 2006.

In this brief article, Kosman asserts that John Adams has risen to an iconic status in the likes of Aaron Copland. According to Kosman, these two composers define the American musical tradition of their generations in an unparalleled way that no other American composer could—Kosman quibbles over Samuel Barber's *genteel* music, Charles Ives's ornery and disruptive music, Leonard Bernstein's stylistic inconsistencies, and Elliott Carter's cacophonic sounds. For Kosman, Adams's orchestral triptych *My Father Knew Charles Ives* puts a stamp on Adams as the foremost American composer of our time for its attempt to express the indigenous American musical tradition.

214. Kozinn, Allan. "Beyond Minimalism: The Later Works of John Adams." *The New York Times* (March 23, 2005). www.nytimes.com/2005/03/23/arts/music/beyond-minimalism-the-later-works-of-john-adams.html.

Kozinn is one of the music critics who purport that Adams's recent works do not adhere to strict minimalist principles. According to Kozinn, Adams's works from 1992 onwards show a different trend where repetitive patterns peek through sporadically. The composer's music has become one of inclusion of myriad styles. Adams incorporates influences from jazz, blues, rock music, and even cartoon soundtracks. One might question what a postminimalist aesthetic entails, and whether it is inclusive of other styles as composers Michael Torke and Arvo Pärt have synthesized their own inclusive musical languages. Another assumption readers might consider is whether dissonance and chromaticism exclude musical works from the minimalist camp, as Kozinn believes.

215.   _____. "Summing Up John Adams at Midcareer." *The New York Times* (November 28, 1999). www.nytimes.com/1999/11/28/arts/summing-up-john-adams-at-midcareer.html.

Kozinn reflects on Adams's career shortly after the release of *The John Adams Earbox* 10-CD collection on the Nonesuch label. He states that Adams's early works changed the course of minimalism through the integration of chromaticism and gesture to create a more expressive style. Kozinn finds "peculiar parallels" between Copland and Adams; in fact, he devotes nearly the entire article to this point—Adams has similarly found an affinity for Copland. Both composers worked in academic styles before discovering their more popular American sound. Adams's *Christian Zeal and Activity* bears a "striking resemblance to the devotional orchestral fabric of Copland's 'Lincoln Portrait'." Both composers grew restless with their native musical styles. For a time Copland explored Neo-Classicism and serialism while revisiting his folk influences in passing. In the same token, Kozinn finds parallels of harmonic density between Adams's *Harmonium* and Ligeti's works. Additionally, the Violin Concerto eschews early minimalist rigidity for a greater affinity towards counterpoint. Adams and Copland's connection to the vernacular merits attention as well. Copland paints his image of America with hymns and folk tunes. Similarly, references to pop and rock abound in Adams's works. From a larger perspective, Kozinn asserts that the link between these two composers is a neo-Romantic aesthetic. In the latter portion of his article, Kozinn presents Adams's oeuvre as a tour de force, with each work contributing to the ongoing ingenuity found in his music. *Eros Piano*, for instance, is portrayed as a bridge that gave way to a new harmonic style with harmonizations reminiscent of Bill Evans's piano voicings.

216.   Lipman, Samuel. "The Second Death of Klinghoffer." *Commentary* 92, no. 5 (1991): 46–9.

Lipman begins his review with one of the most detailed historical accounts of the *Achille Lauro* cruise ship hijacking that led to the death of Leon Klinghoffer. Before embarking on a critical review of Adams's *Klinghoffer* opera, Lipman familiarizes readers with the opera's collaborators. He characterizes Adams's first opera in a negative light as incidental music, subpar to the libretto. Lipman asserts that the world reaction of the current event as depicted in the news was overshadowed in Adams's opera. He purports that the real Klinghoffer stood as a heroic symbol for the millions of victims from the Holocaust. Lipman believes the collaborators had the mindset of creating a trendy and "cutting-edge" opera, which meant taking a neutral stance toward the Israeli-Palestinian conflict, and for this reason, the opera is not titled *The Murder of Klinghoffer*. Lipman offers disparaging remarks for every aspect of Adams's opera, from the production to the libretto and music. The critic opines that Adams's compositional abilities are limited to four musical techniques, which, in the end, render the music to be utilitarian. Lipman's criticisms are not reserved for Adams and his collaborators alone, as he states that minimalism is capable of expressing only a single mood and is not able to stand on its own without text. While there are parallels between Lipman and Richard Taruskin's reviews, the former exceeds the limits of subject matter to question the validity of the minimalist aesthetic.

217. Page, Tim. "Nixon in China." *Newsday* (March 29, 1988). Reprinted in *The John Adams Reader: Essential Writings on an American Composer*, ed. Thomas May, 294–6. Pompton Plains: Amadeus, 2006.

Page writes a candid review of *Nixon in China* shortly after its world premiere. Music critics' initial responses to the opera were often scathing, and portions of Page's writing reveal the harsh musical environment. Page purports that the opera transformed Kissinger into a "venal, jabbering, opportunistic buffoon" (295). Aside from this statement, Page's commentary is more balanced than the majority of early reviews. Page's critique is also informative regarding changes made to the opera following the New York production. The second act was bisected to provide an intermission before the meditative finale, which now forms part of Act III. This new method of delivery proved more pleasing for the collaborators, who chose to make the revision permanent.

218. Rich, Alan. "Born Again (Film of *The Death of Klinghoffer*)." *LA Weekly* (November 10, 2003). Reprinted in *The John Adams Reader: Essential Writings on an American Composer*, ed. Thomas May, 340–2. Pompton Plains: Amadeus, 2006.

The late Alan Rich discusses director Penny Woolcock's 2003 film adaptation of Adams's *The Death of Klinghoffer*. Rich dispels any doubts about his beliefs of the opera's place in contemporary music: "Nobody of consequence has ever challenged the intense *musical* power of John Adams's opera" (340). The film was created with the help of Adams himself around the time of the September 11 terrorist attack. This film revives the event that led to the death of Leon Klinghoffer, though it should be noted it is not the first film that attempts to recreate the past. Prior to the opera itself, director Robert L. Collins released his film *The Hijacking of the Achille Lauro* in 1989 that recounts how the hijacking unfolded in 1985. Woolcock's version is drawn directly from Adams's opera, including the music, which Adams conducts himself. Rich gives the film favorable ratings, and purports that even though Adams's score has been drastically reworked, the fluidity of the opera is managed brilliantly in the film. Viewers might contemplate what has compelled Adams to recreate his opera in a different medium, one that has the power to reach mainstream media in a manner foreign to today's opera, in spite of all the criticism and backlash the composer and librettist have received over the years. If *Nixon in China* put Adams on the international map, then *Klinghoffer* assured his place as one of the great composers of our time. Woolcock's film further solidifies Adams as one of the foremost, forward-thinking composers today.

219.   ____. "Learning to Love the Bomb (*Doctor Atomic*)." *LA Weekly* (October 14, 2005). Reprinted in *The John Adams Reader: Essential Writings on an American Composer*, ed. Thomas May, 382–5. Pompton Plains: Amadeus, 2006.

Rich lauds Adams's latest achievement of *Doctor Atomic* shortly after its world premiere. As a preamble to discussing the work, Rich contextualizes Adams's operatic works in light of contemporary classical music, asserting that American opera has risen to a golden age thanks to Adams. Rich states that Adams's opera brings issues of morality and ideals to the forefront. He praises the manner in which Peter Sellars created the libretto by compiling text from military and scientific notes and numerous other sources. In the music and libretto, Rich detects traces of Wagner's *Parsifal* in its treatment of the troubled genius, mystic, and hero. Characters in the opera take shape as real people, and not superficial facades of their true selves: Kitty is an alcoholic, and her text draws solace from Muriel Rukeyser's poetry, while Robert gets lost in the poetry of John Donne. Concerning the subject matter of the opera, Rich hails it as timeless and Adams's setting of the libretto deeply penetrates the troubled souls of his characters. Rich believes *Doctor Atomic* is the culminating result of his earlier operas.

220.   ____. "Life as Music: John Adams Goes Public." *LA Weekly* (October 3, 2003). Reprinted in *The John Adams Reader: Essential Writings on an American Composer*, ed. Thomas May, 63–6. Pompton Plains: Amadeus, 2006.

Rich engages with Adams's *On the Transmigration of Souls* and *The Dharma at Big Sur*, contextualizing the works with passages from an interview with the composer. Adams regards both of these recent works as large public pieces. Numerous other sources detail the history behind the making of *On the Transmigration of Souls*—the content included here is no different. Regarding *The Dharma at Big Sur*, Adams reveals that Lou Harrison's *Concerto in Slendro* served as a model for integrating Indonesian scales and rhythms—this is also detailed in Adams's official website, to some extent.

221.   ____. "Mischief (*Grand Pianola Music*)." *LA Weekly* (July 30, 2004). Reprinted in *The John Adams Reader: Essential Writings on an American Composer*, ed. Thomas May, 286–7. Pompton Plains: Amadeus, 2006.

Rich recounts a 2004 performance of *Grand Pianola Music* at the Hollywood Bowl. Adams's piano concerto was programmed right after Beethoven's "Emperor" Concerto, which was influential in the making of the former. Impressions of the work on the audience were mixed. Rich's neighbors at the next box at the Bowl perceived Adams's concerto to be crude in comparison to Beethoven's, and while they both contain sections that emphasize E-flat major arpeggios, the result is markedly different. Rich also recalls being at the premiere of *Grand Pianola Music* in San Francisco, where the audience response was thrilling, and a year later in New York, where the audience strongly disliked the work. Rich concludes his article stating, "[t]here's still work to be done" in order to change the average concertgoer's impressions about a minimalist composer such as Adams and regard him as part of the same historical canon as Beethoven (287).

222.   ____. "Something to Say (Violin Concerto)." *LA Weekly* (November 9, 2004). Reprinted in *The John Adams Reader: Essential Writings on an American Composer*, ed. Thomas May, 343–4. Pompton Plains: Amadeus, 2006.

Rich offers a critique of violinist Leila Josefowicz's performance of Adams's Violin Concerto at the Walt Disney Concert Hall. Leila Josefowicz is regarded as a proponent of Adams's music and that of other contemporary composers. Rich gives a glowing review and discusses the piece in brief, deriving material from Adams's program notes. Rich compares Josefowicz's performance to Gidon Kremer's recording of the concerto, performed with the London Symphony Orchestra under the direction of Kent Nagano.

223.   Roca, Octavio. "N.Y. City Ballet, John Adams Make a Dazzling Team." *San Francisco Chronicle* (June 8, 1995). www.sfgate.com/entertainment/article/N-Y-City-Ballet-John-Adams-Make-A-Dazzling-Team-3031227.php.

San Francisco Chronicle dance critic Roca details how Peter Martins, director and resident choreographer of the City Ballet, created a major new American ballet based on Adams's Violin Concerto. Roca highlights key moments of the concerto along with Martin's choreography and describes the orchestral tumult of the first movement where two men dance in counterpoint to the emotion of Adams's concerto. Roca also elaborates on Martin's choreography for the Adagio movement and the finale.

224.   Rockwell, John. "From an Episode of Terrorism, Adams's *Death of Klinghoffer*." *The New York Times* (March 21, 1991). Reprinted in *The John Adams Reader: Essential Writings on an American Composer*, ed. Thomas May, 313–16. Pompton Plains: Amadeus, 2006.

Following the Brussels premiere of *The Death of Klinghoffer*, Rockwell offers his perspective on the opera. Rockwell highlights aspects of the opera that have been discussed in detail by other writers. First, Adams's musical style transforms Reich's minimalist techniques into a dramatic form with the integration of neo-Romantic lyricism. Second, Adams's score blends conventional and electronic instruments, along with amplification of the singers, which, at its best, creates new sound colors, and at its worst, muddles textures. In Rockwell's estimation, Sellars's "half-realized ideas" are inadequate in Act I, Mark Morris's choreography is incongruously formalistic, and Adams's music fails to articulate English words with clarity (315). The author reviews Act II more favorably, from the drama to the vivid acting of *Klinghoffer* and two antagonists. Rockwell's qualms about the opening of the opera do not seem all that significant for the author, remarking in his last paragraph that a better production of the opera could turn into standing ovations.

225.   Ross, Alex. "COUNTDOWN: John Adams and Peter Sellars Create an Atomic Opera." *The New Yorker* (September 25, 2005). www.newyorker.com/magazine/2005/10/03/countdown-4.

Ross promotes the upcoming world premiere of Adams's *Doctor Atomic* in San Francisco. He elaborates on the daunting undertaking of premiering the opera with its extensive list of collaborators, ranging from choreographer, set designer, costume designer, lighting designer, and others, totaling about five hundred people involved in the production. Ross details the specific work required of each designer in fulfilling their task. He acquaints readers with Pamela Rosenberg, who was instrumental in pitching the topic of an Oppenheimer opera and commissioning the work with the San Francisco Opera. The author explores Sellars's experience with opera, going back to his undergraduate thesis on the Russian theater director Vsevolod Meyerhold and his interest in avant-garde theater and Konstantin Stanislavsky's psychological naturalism. Ross notes that Sellars shuns facile depictions of good versus evil in his portrayal of operatic characters—Adams shares the same ideology, as demonstrated in *Nixon in China* and *The Death of Klinghoffer*. Ross details Sellars's creation of the libretto originating from a number of primary sources. The author describes the partnership between Adams and Sellars as one of respect for each other's craft, though not always in agreement. Ross cites Sellars, who calls attention to the passage of time in the opera and the doomsday countdown at its conclusion. Sellars elaborates on the end of the opera, emphasizing that inside every minute is a universe. Sellars elevates *Doctor Atomic* to classics such as *Götterdämmerung*, though geared for modern audiences.

Delving into some analytical inquiry, Ross opines that Adams's A-major and F-minor polyharmony throughout the opera foreshadows the catastrophic conclusion. Ross describes Adams's daily compositional routine in the making of this opera. To this day, Adams still composes on music staff paper, though he concurrently works out compositional problems with computer software. Yet unlike his earlier works, Adams did not make an initial piano sketch. Ross touches on musical influences for this opera. One noteworthy connection is the music of Edgard Varèse. By coincidence, Ross notes that some of the physicists from the Manhattan Project entertained themselves with a recording from Varèse's *Ionization*. Other models include Stravinsky's *Symphony of Psalms* and the harmonic language from his own *Harmonielehre* period. Ross devotes the latter portion of his article to give a detailed account of the most dramatic and noteworthy events of the opera.

226.   ____. "The Dark Side of the Gold Rush: John Adams's New Opera, *Girls of the Golden West*, Is an Assault on American Mythology." *The New Yorker* (December 4, 2017). www.newyorker.com/magazine/2017/12/11/the-dark-side-of-the-gold-rush.

In anticipation of Adams's *Girls of the Golden West* premiere, Ross writes a piece that explores the opera and its connection to American mythology. The collaborators sought to address provocative subjects as they pertain to the California Gold Rush, yet without romanticizing the subject matter. Readers will note the collaborators continue their documentary style of libretto writing, which appeals to historically oriented audiences. Ross critiques the opera as a work of art, yet states it is uneven in treatment, perhaps too long, and would have more impact in trimmer form. The moment in question for Ross is Act I, which attempts to present an unconventional fantasy of gold-rush life. Ross considers the opera a good first draft, perhaps under the false pretext that all of Adams's operas are subject to extensive revision in the *Klinghoffer* manner. Ross touches on several other items: he introduces and praises members of the cast and discusses Adams's musical style for setting this new opera as bearing remnants of *Nixon in China*.

227.   _____. "Dept. of Raw Nerves: Hijack Opera Scuttled." *The New Yorker* (November 19, 2001). Reprinted in *The John Adams Reader: Essential Writings on an American Composer*, ed. Thomas May, 328–30. Pompton Plains: Amadeus, 2006.

Ross discusses *Boston Symphony Orchestra*'s 2001 cancellation of select numbers from *The Death of Klinghoffer* for fear that audiences would be "too fragile" following the 9/11 terrorist attack (328). Meanwhile, Ross notes the San Francisco Symphony was performing Berlioz's *Symphonie Fantastique*, a work portraying a violent execution. Adams views this as a double standard and does not understand why the Boston Symphony would buckle under pressure. We learn that one of the reasons for its cancellation had to do with the fact that a member of the Tanglewood Festival Chorus—set to perform with the Boston Symphony—had been killed in the attack. Adams was not swayed by the orchestra's reasons for canceling the performance.

228.   _____. "The Harmonist." *The New Yorker* (January 8, 2001). Reprinted in *The John Adams Reader: Essential Writings on an American Composer*, ed. Thomas May, 29–44. Pompton Plains: Amadeus, 2006.

Ross's article, written shortly after his visit to Adams's home, offers a good introduction to Adams's musical style, geared for readers largely unacquainted with the composer. Ross considers Adams a romantic minimalist for having "mapped fragments of romantic harmony onto the electric grid of minimalism" (36). Ross gives readers a glimpse of Adams's thoughts on the reception of several of his large works: *Harmonielehre*, *Nixon in China*, *Naive and Sentimental Music*, and *El Niño*. Adams's tonal approach in *Harmonielehre* and *Grand Pianola Music* also receives attention. Speaking on the compositional process, Adams discusses his attention to creating musical spaces with tonal harmonies and his penchant for writing large minimalist structures. Adams recounts his experiences as a graduate student and the impact of early minimalists on his compositional development. The composer highlights the significance of early works like *Harmonielehre* in breaking away from the prevailing compositional style stemming from the East Coast musical establishment.

229.   Rothstein, Edward. "Early Works." *The New Republic* (December 2, 1985). Reprinted in *The John Adams Reader: Essential Writings on an American Composer*, ed. Thomas May, 282–5. Pompton Plains: Amadeus, 2006.

Rothstein introduces readers to Adams's *Harmonielehre*, a newly premiered work when this author wrote his article. Rothstein quotes some background information directly from the composer. The work is not a commentary on Schoenberg's harmony treatise, but rather a displaying of Adams's harmonic vocabulary. Rothstein's depiction of Adams's style is typical of writers during the 1980s. As the author states, "Mr. Adams's unique combination of bad taste and bad faith has undermined both traditions," he clearly reveals his bias in thwarting the pure kind of minimalism that Reich and his contemporaries relied upon (283). Rothstein continues his harsh criticism, characterizing *Grand Pianola Music* as meaningless and grotesque. He laments what he considers as the demise of minimalism brought on by Adams himself. Yet in the midst of his misguided criticism, he implicitly stumbles on a wonderful assertion that Adams is a new kind of minimalist—which he nevertheless fears. It is this style of *perverse* minimalism that eventually came to be known as postminimalism, a natural continuum from the original yet without its stubbornness. Sadly, Rothstein, who longed for the early days of this musical style, concludes in his article that Adams has used minimalism as a "tool in his grab bag of clichés, a cover for an absence of thought, a gesture toward the avant-garde in music that is fundamentally directionless" (285).

230.   _____. "Nixon in China." *The New Republic* (January 4, 1988). Reprinted in *The John Adams Reader: Essential Writings on an American Composer*, ed. Thomas May, 288–93. Pompton Plains: Amadeus, 2006.

Shortly after the world premiere of *Nixon in China*, Rothstein predicts that Adams's opera would hold an important place in contemporary music. The author opines Adams's opera is, thematically speaking, a kind of sequel to Glass's *Satyagraha*. Glass's opera is a heroic one about Gandhi, in which the scenes have a counterpart in the 1960s counterculture, and Adams's *Nixon* portrays a meeting of its counterculture's villains and some of its heroes. Rothstein believes that Adams depicted the American protagonists as demonic and buffoonish villains. Listening to Adams discuss the opera in interviews, I perceive that Adams is interested in the complex character of Nixon and showing the rise and fall of people in power such as the president, rather than presenting an oversimplified portrayal of good-versus-evil polarities. It is Rothstein's contention that the result of the individual approaches by Goodman, Adams, and Sellars produces a "polymorphously perverse" opera (292). In summary, Rothstein believes that the depiction of these characters is in the spirit of the avant-garde rather than an attempt at accurate portrayal. Henry Kissinger's memoirs paint a different light on these characters. Of Chairman Mao, he knew the revolution destroyed the country, killing millions, overturning institutions, and purging the Party. To portray Mao in this way would result in a tragic, rather than postmodern opera.

231.   _____. "Seeking Symmetry Between Palestinians and Jews." Reprinted in *The John Adams Reader: Essential Writings on an American Composer*, ed. Thomas May, 317–20. Pompton Plains: Amadeus, 2006.

Rothstein offers a review of *The Death of Klinghoffer* shortly after the New York premiere. The author purports that the central themes from this opera go beyond politics. Rothstein's impressions of Adams's musical setting are not favorable, stating that the music is seriously limited in range. He quibbles over musical processes such as ostinatos, part of the minimalist aesthetic, as ominous murmurings. He characterizes the music as "atmospheric or emotionally elementary, while the text is set in so unmusical a fashion that the surtitles are required to decipher it" (318). Rothstein's position on the Klinghoffer debate is not entirely clear. On the periphery, his statement "who could tell from this work just what the Jewish side really is" expresses his opinion as a lopsided treatment of Arabs and Jews (319). I suspect Rothstein's critique may have influenced subsequent writers to follow up with more biting reviews, such as Richard Taruskin's condemnation piece. Rothstein also provides a critique of the libretto, declaring that "ideas are undeveloped, cryptic passages are chanted, mixed metaphors created, [and] references left unclear" (319). Rothstein concludes that the libretto is incoherent and the score unconvincing, resulting in a work that only poses as daringly breaking new ground.

232.   Ruhe, Pierre. "Composer Captures Essence of Today." *The Atlanta Journal-Constitution* (May 23, 2003). Reprinted in *The John Adams Reader: Essential Writings on an American Composer*, ed. Thomas May, 53–8. Pompton Plains: Amadeus, 2006.

Ruhe surveys Adams's works, providing background and anecdotal information from Adams's composition teacher David Del Tredici. Adams's teacher recalls his impressions of his student while at Harvard. Ruhe begins his survey exploring Adams's most recent large-scale work (at the time), *El Niño*. As told by Adams, the model for *El Niño* was Handel's *Messiah*, though Adams's own account of the nativity story is more diverse, encompassing writings from the Gospels, Apocryphal Tales, and poems by Latin American women writers about childbirth. Other works are discussed in brief, supported by relevant information from Adams's program notes.

233.   Schiff, David. "Memory Spaces (*On the Transmigration of Souls*) (2002)." *The Atlantic* (April 2003). Reprinted in *The John Adams Reader: Essential Writings on an American Composer*, ed. Thomas May, 189–95. Pompton Plains: Amadeus, 2006.

Schiff describes Adams as the most influential and aesthetically ambitious composer of our time. The composer's achievements transformed the symphony orchestra into the twenty-first century. According to Schiff, Adams emphasizes the bright upper register to make an ensemble of mostly acoustic instruments sound electronically synthesized. Schiff offers a brief biography before exploring Adams's *On the Transmigration of Souls*. The manner in which the author situates Adams's style within contemporary music and culture is generally useful, but he also reveals some generalizations about minimalism that are detrimental to readers' understanding of Adams's style, stating that Adams is a "master of rhythm, texture, and color but not a melodist" (191). Works such as *Nixon in China* and the Violin Concerto are propelled by a foreground melodic iteration and development; thus, Schiff's assessment is misleading. Nevertheless, Schiff raises some interesting points about Adams's *Transmigration*. First, Adams redefines "the relation of music to non-music and of the concert hall to everyday life" (192). Schiff notes that *Transmigration* mixes sound elements in a way that seems foreign to classical music and more akin to the movie theater experience. Second, he asserts that *Transmigration* builds on Ives's vision from his work "From Hanover Square North, at the End of a Tragic Day, the Voice of the People Again Arose" (193). Following this connection between the two composers, Schiff gives a digest version of the work itself, from the opening sound collage to the use of taped recordings, the chorus parts, and the orchestra's eruptions throughout *Transmigration*.

234.   Schmid, Rebecca. "John Adams on How to Conduct Yourself." *The Financial Times* (September 23, 2016). www.ft.com/content/aabfad88-7f25-11e6-8e50-8ec15fb462f4.

Schmid remarks that Adams has become the first composer-in-residence of the Berliner Philharmoniker since 1998. During this time, Adams was preparing a concert to kick off his tenure with this orchestra, featuring many of his musical works and the German premiere of *Scheherazade.2*. Adams discusses the importance of conducting for a composer's creative process and its influence on his own musical works. Schmid notes a recurring theme in Adams's compositions, which portray women as heroines challenged by unique circumstances, as in *Scheherazade.2*, but also other compositions like the telling of the nativity from Mary's perspective in *El Niño*, or his opera *Girls of the Golden West*. Remarking on his compositional career, Adams claims that he is neither a neo-Romantic nor a postminimalist composer because the labels disparage half of his output, which he deems to be from neither camp. The last topic Schmid and Adams discuss concerns his 2012 composition for string quartet and orchestra *Absolute Jest*. Reflecting on the compositional process in *Absolute Jest*, Adams explains that he "manipulated fragments from Beethoven's late string quartets through a software program" as an homage to his predecessor.

235.   Seibert, Brian. "Dance This Week: 'Available Light' and Louise Lecavalier." *The New York Times* (September 8, 2015). www.nytimes.com/2015/09/08/arts/dance/dance-this-week-available-light-and-louise-lecavalier.html.

Seibert announces the 2015 revival of Adams's 1983 collaboration "Available Light," with multiple upcoming performances across the U.S. and Europe. The author highlights the significance of this collaboration from the perspective of Lucinda Childs's choreography and its impact on modern dance.

236.   Sheridan, Molly. "San Francisco Symphony and John Adams Embark on 10-Year Plan." *NewMusicBox* (July 1, 2001). https://nmbx.newmusicusa.org/San-Francisco-Symphony-and-John-Adams-Embark-on-10year-Plan.

Sheridan writes a news article following the San Francisco Symphony's announcement of a ten-year commission with John Adams that will culminate with the orchestra's 100th season. The announcement coincides with the twentieth anniversary of the world premiere of *Harmonium*, which also was commissioned by the San Francisco Symphony. In the remainder of her article, Sheridan highlights Adams's premieres and commissions with this orchestra.

237.   Sisario, Ben. "At Nonesuch Records, Star Treatment for a Boss Who Plays." *The New York Times* (March 30, 2017). www.nytimes.com/2017/03/30/arts/music/robert-hurwitz-nonesuch-celebration.html.

Sisario's article reflects on Robert Hurwitz's career as president of Nonesuch Records. Hurwitz has been an instrumental figure in the promotion of Adams's works through numerous recordings. Adams has composed and dedicated his most recent piano solo piece, *I Still Play*, to Hurwitz to memorialize their friendship and as a farewell following his retirement. Along with this tribute, Adams has organized a concert in Hurwitz's honor which includes other pieces composed for the occasion by composers Laurie Anderson, Louis Andriessen, Philip Glass, Brad Mehldau, Randy Newman, Steve Reich, and others.

238.   Stayton, Richard. "The Trickster of Modern Music: Composer John Adams Keeps Reinventing Himself, to Wilder and Wilder Applause." *Los Angeles Times* (June 16, 1991). www.latimes.com/archives/la-xpm-1991-06-16-tm-1335-story.html.

Stayton visits Adams's home and writes his account about the composer shortly after the premiere of his second opera, *The Death of Klinghoffer*. Stayton opines that Klinghoffer's death is a ritualized crucifixion, symbolic of the Gospel in the sense that the main protagonist is an innocent man who dies for our sins. Even at this point in Adams's career, the composer was uneasy with the categorization of his works as minimalist. Adams criticizes the contemporary obsession for musical purity because it brings about sterility. The composer Fred Myrow comments on Adams's compositional achievements; namely, he adopted minimalist techniques yet formed a new offshoot with a "more ambitious musical architecture than Philip Glass." As a byproduct of forging his new path, Adams broke away from the influential European composers of the time, including Berio, Boulez, and Stockhausen.

239.   Swed, Mark. "Adams's Twentieth Century Rolls—and Rocks (*Century Rolls*)." *Los Angeles Times* (February 5, 2001). Reprinted in *The John Adams Reader: Essential Writings on an American Composer*, ed. Thomas May, 355–8. Pompton Plains: Amadeus, 2006.

Swed begins his review of Adams's piano concerto *Century Rolls* by distinguishing between popular music and contemporary classical music, which is a topic Adams often discusses during interviews. His definition is refutable at best: pop music speaks in a common tongue about the present, whereas contemporary classical music has a larger view of the past and is more complex. The author segues to Adams's love for three jazzy piano concertos—by Ravel, Gershwin, and Copland—and their influence in his own work. Another well-documented motivation for *Century Rolls* is piano rolls themselves, which are mechanical in nature, and Swed makes an association with the negative stereotype of the minimalist style as broken-record music. Swed also discusses several of Adams's selections from *Nixon in China* he compiled called "The Nixon Tapes." This suite contains the opening scene of the opera, Pat Nixon's aria from the second act, and the banquet and toasts by Chou En-lai and Nixon. Swed turns to performances of Adams's works, noting that in the *Los Angeles Philharmonic* performance he attended, the balance between soloists and the orchestra needed fine-tuning. Swed favors conductors Kent Nagano, Esa-Pekka Salonen, and Michael Tilson Thomas as interpreters of Adams's music above the composer himself.

240.   ____. "After 32 Years, 'Available Light' Brighter Than Ever." *Los Angeles Times* (June 7, 2015). www.latimes.com/entertainment/la-et-cm-available-light-review-20150608-column.html.

Swed discusses the revival of *Available Light*, a collaboration between composer John Adams, choreographer Lucinda Childs, and architect Frank Gehry. After a long hiatus, this fifty-minute music and dance work was performed in June 2015 to celebrate The Music Center's 50th anniversary. Swed remarks that Adams's scoring, titled *Light Over Water*, was composed during Adams's Jungian period. Swed reflects on the negative reception the work received after its premiere in 1983 but hopes to correct people's misconceptions of the work, calling it a brilliant merging of dance, music, and stage setting and design.

241.   ____. "Bigger Proves Better in Adams's Grandiose World (*Naive and Sentimental Music*)." *Los Angeles Times* (February 22, 1999). Reprinted in *The John Adams Reader: Essential Writings on an American Composer*, ed. Thomas May, 359–61. Pompton Plains: Amadeus, 2006.

Swed reviews the world premiere of Adams's *Naive and Sentimental Music* performed with the Los Angeles Philharmonic. He discusses the title of the work as it relates to Adams's "dual personalities," the serious versus the trickster, and notes that the musical schizophrenia has finally healed. Swed claims that Adams gives us more of everything in this orchestral symphony: jazz becomes jazzier, melancholy more devastating, and rhythmic energy more obsessive. I find Swed's review to be overly general and highly subjective. Readers are left to ponder what aspects of the symphony seem jazzier than earlier works such as *Lollapalooza*, and how is Adams's rhythmic treatment more obsessive than in *Fearful Symmetries*, a piece rhythmically driven by the repetition of harmonies and symmetrical phrase structures?

242.   ____. "John Adams' 'Ceiling/Sky' Remains Earthbound." *Los Angeles Times* (August 25, 2014). www.latimes.com/entertainment/arts/classical/la-et-cm-ceiling-sky-review-20140825-column.html.

Looking back at Adams's 1995 opera/musical *I Was Looking at the Ceiling and Then I Saw the Sky*, Swed purports it provides social commentary as a worldly and spiritual response to the 1992 Los Angeles riots and the 1994 Northridge earthquake. Swed relates the events that inspired *Ceiling/Sky* to today's unrest with natural disasters and the recent violence that ensued in Ferguson, Missouri following a police brutality verdict in 2014. Swed believes this is one way in which a 90s musical work can seem pertinent in today's society. This critic's review is generally positive, though he clearly states Adams's work could stand a revision, specifically pertaining to the unbalance of proportions between the long first act and the significantly shorter second act. As a final thought, Swed suggests that Adams's *Ceiling/Sky* suggests a way forward for society and for Broadway, but neither one has chosen to listen.

243.   ____. "On Top, But Ever the Risk-Taker." *Los Angeles Times* (January 28, 2001). Reprinted in *The John Adams Reader: Essential Writings on an American Composer*, ed. Thomas May, 45–52. Pompton Plains: Amadeus, 2006.

Swed reflects on Adams's compositional career and the significance of his works in today's classical world. He claims that Adams receives more attention in the press than any other contemporary composer, his music is in highest demands for performances and recordings, his works generate great anticipation at home and abroad, and his works have earned him great respect from professionals and music lovers alike. Swed also celebrates other successes: *Century Rolls* was receiving its Los Angeles premiere during this time, his symphony *Naive and Sentimental Music* marked a Beethovenian triumph at the close of the millennium, and his oratorio *El Niño* aroused a great deal of attention for its female perspective on the nativity story. Speaking on the controversial nature of Adams's operatic works, Swed purports that Adams and his collaborators do not seek controversy for its own sake; rather, Adams's operas raise important issues of social relevance today. Towards the end of his piece, Swed explores Adams's use of technology and microphone amplification in his operatic works.

244.   ____. "Rebirth of a Savior in *El Niño*." *Los Angeles Times* (January 13, 2001). Reprinted in *The John Adams Reader: Essential Writings on an American Composer*, ed. Thomas May, 362–4. Pompton Plains: Amadeus, 2006.

A month following the world premiere of *El Niño* in Paris, and just two days after the North American premiere in San Francisco, Swed writes his review of Adams's *El Niño*. As is known, Adams's oratorio *El Niño* depicts the birth of Christ in a new way. Sellars recorded a silent film depicting Los Angeles street life, which runs during the entire performance. Swed posits the message of Adams's work is truly novel, and the message is an attempt to unite people by portraying the birth of Christ not as a religious miracle but rather a biological one. Swed highly praises Adams's music, which is modeled after Handel's *Messiah*. Swed assures readers that the blend and unity of texts as diverse as the Bible, Gnostic sources, Latin American poetry, and texts by Hildegard von Bingen are what make Adams's musical style so effective. This critic describes Adams's music as rich, complex, rolling, forceful, and eager for a magnificent climax. Regarding the quality of the work, Swed hails *El Niño* as Adams's newest great hit, having catchier tones and spikier rhythms than seen in earlier works—this critic has a natural tendency to praise Adams's latest opuses over previously composed works.

245.   ____. "Seeking Answers in an Opera." *Los Angeles Times* (October 7, 2001).
        Reprinted in *The John Adams Reader: Essential Writings on an American Com-*
        poser, ed. Thomas May, 321–7. Pompton Plains: Amadeus, 2006.

        Mark Swed reflects on Adams's opera *The Death of Klinghoffer* ten years after its
        premiere. Swed has written numerous favorable reviews of Adams's music in the
        Los Angeles Times, even before Adams became a household name in the music
        world. He sums up his opinion on *Klinghoffer's* treatment of terrorism, stating
        that the opera neither supports terrorism nor apologizes for it, but it asks that
        listeners identify with emotions that drive the actions we despise. Swed remains
        staunch in his opinion that the opera does not side with terrorism: one only has
        to witness Marilyn's rage over the death of her husband. The beauty of the music
        is unparalleled, according to the writer.

        Swed traces the events that may have led to the opera's controversy. The times
        were charged by the recent hijacking of the *Achille Lauro*, and the premiere took
        place under tight security in Brussels a week after the end of the Gulf War. Pro-
        tests came from opposite ends of the spectrum: some claimed it was a Zionist
        plot, while others called it unashamedly pro-Palestinian. Adams's own thoughts
        on the reception of his work reveal he is conflicted by people's displeasure yet
        believes audiences must grapple with art on its own terms. Interestingly enough,
        nobody protested the two film versions of the hijacking because the terrorists
        were portrayed as one-dimensional "comic-book villains" (324). One of the
        reasons American opera companies shied away from performances of Adams's
        opera is that, unlike their European counterparts, they rely heavily on private
        funding.

246.   Taruskin, Richard. "Music's Dangers and the Case for Control." *The New York*
        Times (December 9, 2001). Reprinted in *The John Adams Reader: Essential Writ-*
        ings on an American Composer, ed. Thomas May, 331–9. Pompton Plains: Ama-
        deus, 2006.

        Taruskin writes a long-drawn introduction regarding the power of music on
        listeners by recounting prohibitions of music in some religious doctrines and
        tracing writings from the ancient Greeks like Plato's *Republic*. He prepares his
        argument by examining how religions and philosophers have dealt with the doc-
        trine of ethos, and how music affects behavior, character, emotion, and morality.
        After equipping himself with ammunition, he states his argument plainly: for the
        reason that music's effects are seemingly greater than other arts like literature and
        painting, it necessitates control and censorship under special circumstances. He
        cites an example when orchestras and opera companies should use discretion. In
        2001 Maestro Barenboim conducted the music of Wagner in Israel, despite the
        fact it was informally banned and therefore sparked public protest. In the case
        of Adams, Taruskin's analogy does not translate in the same way. While Wagner
        adopted Nazi ideals from Arthur de Gobineau, Adams has never expressed any
        radical ideologies. Taruskin believes that terrorists' motivations should never be
        voiced in art, for doing so romanticizes their actions and makes us sympathetic

to their aims. Taruskin claims that the creators of the opera implicitly acknowledge their guilt by balancing the opening "Chorus of Exiled Palestinians," not with a scene as in the Brussels premiere, but with the "Chorus of Exiled Jews." At the end of his review, Taruskin declares he deplores censorship, but the act of self-control within the arts can be noble.

247.   Tommasini, Anthony. "MUSIC REVIEW: Linking Two Very Different Composers in a Single Recital." *The New York Times* (February 27, 2002). www.nytimes.com/2002/02/27/arts/music-review-linking-two-very-different-composers-in-a-single-recital.html.

Following the world premiere of Adams's piano work *American Berserk* at Carnegie Hall, Tommasini recounts his impressions of the work. The single-movement piano piece is dedicated to the pianist Garrick Ohlsson. The recital program opened with pieces by other composers, followed by Adams's *China Gates* and *American Berserk*. Tommasini considers this latest piano work to be stylistically the opposite of *China Gates*, having "jagged, relentless, harmonically spiky music with out-of-sync lines in block chords happening at once, like those crazy musical collages in Ives." The brevity of this review leaves much to be desired, and readers are urged to refer to Adams's notes on the work directly from his official website.

248.   ____. "Review: John Adams Unveils 'Scheherazade.2,' an Answer to Male Brutality." *The New York Times* (March 27, 2015). www.nytimes.com/2015/03/28/arts/music/review-john-adams-unveils-scheherazade2-an-answer-to-male-brutality.html.

Tommasini published this review the day following the world premiere of Adams's *Scheherazade.2* under the direction of Alan Gilbert with the New York Philharmonic. This music critic commences his review describing the events that inspired Adams to write a concerto devoted to Scheherazade. Adams attended an exhibition in Paris about the history of an *Arabian Nights* collection of folk stories. In conversation with conductor Alan Gilbert, Adams stated he was appalled at the casual brutality towards women in the stories. The theme of the concerto ponders the tales of *Arabian Nights* from the heroine's perspective, written specifically for violinist and proponent of new music Leila Josefowicz. Tommasini describes the role of the soloist in the first movement—entitled "Tale of the Wise Young Woman"—as it "enters playing elegiac lines that keep breaking into skittish flights. Eventually, the violin is set upon by gnashing bursts of jagged chords and a gaggle of crisscrossing orchestral voices, evoking the indignant true believers." In the second movement, entitled "A Long Desire (Love Scene)," Adams suggests Scheherazade's romantic interests could possibly be another woman. Adams's musical depiction of this prospect is characterized by pulsing chords and a "long episode of dreamy, sensual allure." Tommasini writes that the third movement, entitled "Scheherazade and the Men with Beards," suggests that the heroine is charged by the men who bicker over religious doctrine. Tommasini correlates the effect of babbling to the disjunct motion of the musical lines. In the final movement, entitled "Escape, Flight, Sanctuary," the heroine is condemned, but she breaks free. Here the music reaches a searing intensity, with the soloist playing "frenetic eruptions." The author provides a good introductory account of the narrative of Adams's concerto and how the protagonist overcomes her pending doom, though I wish this critic gave additional commentary, whether favorable or negative, concerning his impressions of the work and where it fits within Adams's compositional output.

249.   ____. "Washed in the Sound of Souls in Transit (*On the Transmigration of Souls*)." *The New York Times* (September 21, 2002). Reprinted in *The John Adams Reader: Essential Writings on an American Composer*, ed. Thomas May, 365–7. Pompton Plains: Amadeus, 2006.

In his review of Adams's newly premiered work *On the Transmigration of Souls*, Tommasini captures (and relates) the essence of Adams's newest composition. Adams's intent in writing this work was to create a "memory space" where listeners can reflect on their own thoughts and emotions, transforming the concert hall into a cathedral space for the magnitude and reverence the subject matter demands. Tommasini observes that when the orchestra enters, the string section plays a succession of parallel chords. This chordal planing technique is common for Adams and can be observed in other works, such as the opening measures of the Violin Concerto. According to Tommasini, Adams portrays the solemnity of this music through a subtle mix of tonality with bits of dissonance. To this end, the use of melody is predominantly absent and replaced with spoken leitmotifs using words such as "missing" and "remember." Tommasini avoids writing any discouraging comments and opts for a more neutral and informative review.

250.   Ulrich, Allan. "Scarlett's 'Symmetries' at S.F. Ballet Not the Right Tone." *San Francisco Chronicle* (January 28, 2016). www.sfgate.com/performance/article/ Scarlett-s-Symmetres-at-S-F-Ballet-not-6790449.php.

Ulrich discusses how Adams's *Fearful Symmetries* has served ballet repertoire. Ashley Page's 1995 ballet setting of Adams's composition gained recognition in its performance with London's Royal Ballet. In 2016, choreographer Liam Scarlett introduced his version with the San Francisco Ballet. Ulrich provides an account of Scarlett's rendition, showing displeasure with the performance and claiming that while the choreographer is intimately familiar with the music's structure, he seems oblivious to its tone.

8

Select Video Recordings

251. *John Adams: A Portrait and a Concert of American Music: Music by John Adams, Steve Reich and Conlon Nancarrow.* Produced by Colin Wilson, directed by David Jeffcock. 134 minutes. Arthaus Musik, 2002. DVD 100 323.

This DVD presents a portrait of Adams's life and music as narrated by Amita Dhiri, followed by a recorded concert of Adams's Chamber Symphony and *Gnarly Buttons*. The portrait combines a blend of speech from the narrator and other film footage featuring John Adams, Peter Sellars, Alice Goodman, and Michael Tilson Thomas. The film's portrayal of Adams's life and works is organized into various chapters: (1) Introduction, (2) Childhood/studies at Harvard, (3) Influences on John Adams's Music, (4) *El Niño*, (5) *Nixon in China*, (6) *The Death of Klinghoffer*, (7) and Adams's approach to classical music.

Adams appears as a guest speaker in a classroom, discussing his early days as an aspiring composer and his experiences with avant-garde music while at Harvard University. Speaking on the subject of musical influences, Adams points to his interest in John Cage's philosophies, though eventually, he realized that music indeterminacy was largely inaccessible to listeners. Sometime after graduating from Harvard, Adams recalls a trip to Florence that seemed instrumental to his admiration of minimalist music. Adams noticed the pleasure that Renaissance composers took in the repetition of small, identifiable cells (this account is also told in his autobiography). Adams explains that his early work *Shaker Loops* went against minimalist norms of gradually developing a single idea. His work was "predicated upon minimalist technique" but with "violent changes [and] sudden shocking explosions." Adams elaborates on several other compositions. Concerning what Adams considers one of his "vulgar but full of life" trickster pieces,

Fearful Symmetries, he describes it as a twenty-five-minute-long boogie-woogie. Adams reflects on his artistic aims and desires to create a kind of "mongrel" and impure music that would appeal to listeners today. Later in his discussion, Adams gives a unique insight into Sellars's staging of *El Niño*—viewers can enjoy in more detail. The narrator Dhiri asserts that *Nixon in China* heralded a new genre of opera that relied on contemporary events. Alice Goodman discusses *Nixon in China* and the requisite of grand opera for such a dramatic narrative. Adams claims Nixon's character was set to big-band music circa 1940. Regarding their second collaboration, *The Death of Klinghoffer*, Adams, Sellars, and Goodman maintain that the subject of the opera, as well as their treatment, does not promote anti-Semitic ideology.

252.   *Wonders Are Many: The Making of* Doctor Atomic. Produced and directed by Jon Else. 92 minutes. Docurama Films, 2007. DVD 146 170.

This film by writer, producer, and director Jon Else shows the making of Adams and Sellars's fifth collaboration, *Doctor Atomic*. The film is contextualized in parallel to historical accounts, film footage, and interviews by eminent physicist Freeman Dyson. Jon Else focuses on the science behind the atom bomb, the events that led to the nuclear arms race, and the Manhattan Project. Sellars illustrates his working process of obtaining primary sources and selecting quotations of interest for inclusion in the opera. Adams similarly shows the manner in which he sets the text to music using block harmonies as a sound nucleus. Producer Else devotes a significant portion of the documentary to the rehearsals leading up to the premiere. The portrayal of the final countdown of the atomic bomb is the climax of the entire opera, and this point is emphasized during rehearsals and in Adams's interview clip where he speaks of his compositional process of setting music clocks in different instrument families while simultaneously increasing the tempo for all instrument forces. In sum, the documentary offers an insider's perspective of some important aspects about the opera that include the Trinity site, Oppenheimer's "Batter My Heart" aria, and the final countdown.

9

Other Internet Sources

253. *BBC Music* (July 27, 2016). Accessed May 16, 2019. www.bbc.co.uk/music/artists/94f46f90-f220-458d-acd6-5f14c55ab9b2.

BBC Music devotes online content to the composer John Adams. Users browsing this link can find Adams's biography written by Keith Potter, interviews with the composer, various tracks of Adams's music, and a list of past and upcoming events featuring Adams's works. This BBC page includes an introductory video with Andrew McGregor and John Adams, dated September 3, 2014, honoring the composer for his award as Proms composer and for the premiere of his Saxophone Concerto. McGregor provides an overview of nearly all of Adams's works, together with short music clips, intended for audiences unfamiliar with this body of repertoire. McGregor also surveys multiple recordings, expressing his own preferences between them. The interviewer touches on important musical influences giving rise to Adams's own musical genome, including, but not limited to Wagner, Ives, Riley, Reich, Glass, jazz, and rock.

BBC Music also features its podcast show *Composer of the Week* with host Donald Macleod interviewing John Adams. They discuss Adams's life and works during an hour-long interview, dated April 25, 2014. The host highlights Adams's upbringing and portrays his early minimalist style through *Shaker Loops*. Adams defines the minimalist movement as having a sense of pulsation, a slow harmonic rhythm, and the use of repetition to create large formal structures. The composer himself characterizes his early career in a manner duplicated in other interviews, stating that his early minimalist pieces were more unpredictable and dramatic than that of his minimalist predecessors. Together they discuss an array of Adams's pieces in chronological order, touching on a wide range of subjects:

the history behind the title *American Standard*, the commission of *Harmonium*, the characters in *Nixon in China* (with emphasis on Pat Nixon), the act of caring for the terminally ill in *The Wound-Dresser*, his trickster persona in *Grand Pianola Music* and its outward negation of minimalist norms, his thoughts on the controversy created from *The Death of Klinghoffer* (after nearly thirty years of contemplation on the subject), his role as orchestra conductor for the BBC Symphony Orchestra and the Los Angeles Philharmonic, the background of *John's Book of Alleged Dances*, the mixing of popular culture and highbrowism in the Chamber Symphony, Adams's chromatic sound in the Violin Concerto, the integration of Slonimsky's *Thesaurus of Scales and Melodic Patterns* in recent works, the tradition of American piano concertos in *Century Rolls*, playing between the notes in *The Dharma at Big Sur*, musical beginnings in *My Father Knew Charles Ives*, and memory spaces in *On the Transmigration of Souls*. Internet users seeking additional information can find other interviews with the composer by doing a keyword search on the *BBC Music* website. There is also a 2017 interview titled "John Adams: An American Optimist," where Adams talks with Tom Service about his works, future projects, the current state of professional orchestras, and the role of music in America's political and cultural life today (www.bbc.co.uk/sounds/play/b08bb7qd).

254.   *Boosey & Hawkes*. Accessed May 16, 2019. www.boosey.com/composer/John+Adams.

John Adams's musical scores are under copyright with the British music publisher Boosey & Hawkes. The company owns copyright licenses to his works composed on or after 1987, under the imprint Hendon Music—works composed prior to 1987 are under copyright with G. Schirmer. The webpage devoted to Adams contains a biographical sketch, list of works, select discography, and news items with information on awards, reviews, newly composed works, and upcoming performances. Adams's list of works contains relevant data on their world premieres, along with program notes and scoring requirements for performance needs. Several of the program notes are duplicated from Adams's official website, in part or in full. Many of Adams's scores can be accessed through this website, free of charge, in electronic format. Printed copies are available for purchase or rental for orchestra instrument score parts. Some of the content on the website appears to be original, such as a short video clip and description of the movie *I Am Love*, which is scored to Adams's pre-existing compositions. Alongside the movie preview appears a brief synopsis of the plot and a cue sheet that details specific compositions used in the film (www.boosey.com/podcast/John-Adams-John-Adams-I-Am-Love-with-Tilda-Swinton/12948).

255.   Bruce, David. "John Adams—Modes, Jazz Chords & Slonimsky" (April 29, 2019). Accessed June 15, 2019. www.youtube.com/watch?v=LRCtCB3y7mI.

British composer David Bruce elucidates common compositional techniques found in Adams's works. Early influences such as Steve Reich's *Music for Mallet*

Instruments, Voices and Organ shaped Adams's harmonic progressions and shifts in works such as *Phrygian Gates*. Bruce elaborates on Adams's increasingly intuitive approach to composition in the 80s. Two aspects contribute to this more personal style: (1) the use of oscillating triads for greater forward movement within otherwise static chords and (2) common-tone modulations. Bruce approaches the study of Adams's harmony using a jazz perspective. This approach is meritorious as Adams himself acknowledges studying jazz harmony directly from Miles Davis, Charlie Parker, and John Coltrane, to name a few. According to Bruce, Adams undermines the harmonic structures in the bass register and through embellishing tones. Bruce highlights Adams's greater propensity for dissonance in more recent works, in part resulting from the composer's adoption of Slonimsky's *Thesaurus of Scales and Melodic Patterns*.

256. *CalPerformances*. YouTube. Accessed May 16, 2019. www.youtube.com/user/CalPerformances.

Cal Performances, an organization housed at the University of California, Berkeley, features a series of interviews with John Adams on its YouTube channel. The discussions range from descriptions of his works, including *Light Over Water*, *Shaker Loops*, and his two chamber symphonies, to his experiences conducting music. In his interviews, Adams touches upon various important topics: his early compositional process, collaborating with other artists, and the role of music as a communicative act. He discusses, in brief, *Son of Chamber Symphony* as being more symphonic in nature than its predecessor. The last movement does not bear a title, though Adams notes it might suitably be entitled a dance in the style of a can-can. The influence of Adams's works on film music is undeniable, and in this vein, Adams remarks that *Shaker Loops* was used in the films *Barfly* (1987) and *I Am Love* (2009).

257. Gann, Kyle. "A Course in Postminimalism." Accessed December 22, 2018. www.kylegann.com/AshgatePostminimalism.html.

Gann reproduces an expanded version of his 2013 article "A Technically Definable Stream of Postminimalism, Its Characteristics, and Its Meaning," published in *The Ashgate Research Companion to Minimalist and Postminimalist Music*. Gann's expanded version includes numerous musical excerpts alongside analyses and respective audio clips. As a composer experiencing firsthand the development of the minimalist style in the 1980s and 90s, Gann offers guidance on its origins, style, and development. The author clarifies the origin of the term *postminimalism*, which was coined by *The New York Times* critic John Rockwell as a way to describe Adams's unique musical style. Gann explains that postminimalism embraces an eclectic range of music "beneath its seamlessly even surface." Gann proceeds to discuss a wide array of composers who can be categorized as postminimalist. The latter half of his essay examines common threads among postminimalist composers in their use of repetitive processes, musical quotation, and a continued preoccupation for a reduction of musical materials.

258.   ____. "Fascinating Rhythm: John C. Adams as Metametric Pioneer." Keynote address to the "Inside the (G)earbox: John Adams @ 70" symposium at UCLA (March 4, 2017). Accessed December 21, 2018. www.kylegann.com/Adams-Metametric-Keynote.html.

Composer Kyle Gann publishes this reproduction of his keynote address commemorating Adams's 70th birthday at the 2017 UCLA symposium. Gann reflects on Adams's contributions to the minimalist aesthetic, presenting a selection of works: *China Gates, Shaker Loops, Short Ride in a Fast Machine, Lollapalooza, Naive and Sentimental Music, Gnarly Buttons*, and *The Dharma at Big Sur*. Gann addresses the minimalist process of music loops; specifically, how they go out of sync in Adams's music and how they form part of Adams's rhythmic language. Gann contemplates the origins of using loops, citing Henry Cowell's book *New Musical Resources* as a new theory of rhythm, Joseph Schillinger's theories of rhythm, and Morton Feldman's workings in *Crippled Symmetry*. Gann notes that Adams began juxtaposing loops of different lengths, resulting in a rhythmically complex composite, as early as *China Gates* and subsequently in *Phrygian Gates* and *Shaker Loops*. In *Shaker Loops*, Adams's loops are irregular yet give the aural phenomena or metrical regularity while providing greater rhythm interest—Michael Buchler's 2006 study draws the same conclusions in *Lollapalooza* (see item 274). Gann paints the development of Adams's rhythmic constructs through the manipulation of loops starting with smaller musical mediums (solo and chamber) and culminating with an orchestral treatment in *Lollapalooza*. Adams's experiments with rhythm became the basis in the 1980s and 90s for a musical style Gann calls *totalism*. Examining Adams's harmonic style, Gann observes that in *Naive and Sentimental Music*, Adams's progressions are related by chromatic thirds, a common harmonic syntax of the late Romantic composers. He discusses the applicability of neo-Riemannian musical analysis in these works. The outcome of Adams's looping technique continues to evolve in his twenty-first-century works like *The Dharma at Big Sur*, employing the same preponderance of repeated patterns yet maintaining even less consistency.

259.   *The Kennedy Center.* "An American Tapestry: About the Work." Accessed January 25, 2018. www.kennedy-center.org/artist/composition/4668.

The Kennedy Center features a brief introduction to Adams's music for the film *An American Tapestry*. The film, directed by Gregory Nava and produced by Barbara Martinez-Jitner, released on the Showtime cable channel. John Adams composed over an hour of original music. The Kennedy Center provides a synopsis of the film, which offers personal accounts of Americans from diverse ethnic backgrounds. Adams's music serves to underscore their personal lives and complement the viewpoint that American heritage is founded on the dovetailing of immigrant cultures.

260.   *League of American Orchestras.* Accessed May 16, 2019. www.americanorchestras.org/knowledge-research-innovation/orr-survey.html.

Since the 1970s, the League of American Orchestras has tracked concert programming of professional orchestras and compiled yearly data, which is released in their Orchestra Repertoire Report. Their report ranks John Adams as the most frequently performed living American composer. Adams is ranked number one more consistently than any other composer (in recent years he earned the number one rank for seasons 2004–2005, 2006–2007, 2008–2009, and 2010–2012) and is ranked among the highest for all other years. In addition to the number of performances each year, the report specifies the works and premieres that were performed, together with performance dates, performing orchestra, soloist(s), and conductor.

261. May, Thomas. "Bringing It All Back Home: John Adams at 70" (February 3, 2017). Accessed March 9, 2019. www.sfsymphony.org/Watch-Listen-Learn/Read-Program-Notes/Articles-Interviews/John-Adams-at-70.aspx.

May reflects on Adams's career at 70 and on his long-term relationship with the San Francisco Symphony. Adams has been drawn to this renowned orchestra ever since Edo de Waart became music director in 1977. The following year Adams was appointed new music adviser for the San Francisco Symphony. May offers anecdotal accounts of Adams's early years in San Francisco, which are duplicated in the composer's autobiography. The author speaks about Deborah O'Grady's first encounter with Adams during the inaugural season of Davies Symphony Hall, and he elaborates on their relationship and eventually their marriage and birth of two children. May opines that Adams's music cannot be characterized as minimalism infused with elements from the romantic composers. He opts to describe the defining characteristics of Adams's music: tonality, driving rhythmic energy, pulsation, and a knack for remarkable orchestral colors. May believes Adams seeks to forge new territory with each new composition and will continue as a septuagenarian and beyond.

262. *The Music Sales Group.* "John Adams." Accessed January 6, 2019. www.music salesclassical.com/composer/short-bio/John-Adams.

This publisher's division Music Sales Classical owns rights to all musical scores under the G. Schirmer name. All of Adams's scores predating 1987 are under copyright with The Music Sales Group. The publisher's website contains valuable information regarding Adams's works under the Schirmer label, upcoming performances of these works, a select list of available recordings, and a biography.

263. *National Endowment for the Arts.* Accessed April 7, 2019. www.arts.gov/honors/john-adams.

The National Endowment for the Arts selected Adams for their Opera Honors Award in 2009. Their website features a biography of the composer and various interviews in video and audio format. Adams remarks that the National Endowment for the Arts was instrumental in helping him with the production of *Common Tones in Simple Time.* As a recipient of an NEA award, Adams speaks on the importance of patronage for artists. In an interview, Adams

reflects on his career as composer and conductor, today's political environment, and the profundity of the arts in popular culture (Adams's interview is
available online in the following website: www.arts.gov/video/john-adams-
his-music-contemporary-classical-and-rooted-america).

In another interview, the choreographer Mark Morris speaks on collaborating
with Adams and Sellars. He choreographed the "Red Detachment of Women" for
Nixon in China, the dances used during choruses from *The Death of Klinghoffer*,
and more recently, the *Son of Chamber Symphony*. Morris mentions how the
rhythmic difficulties of Adams's music present interesting challenges for dancers.
NEA Opera also contains an interview with Adams's lifelong artistic collaborator, Peter Sellars. Sellars discusses his early days with Adams, his plans for *Nixon
in China*, and Adams's role in the development of the minimalist style as a dramatic composer.

264.   *Nonesuch Records.* "John Adams." Accessed May 16, 2019. www.nonesuch.com/
       artists/john-adams.

Nonesuch Records has released numerous recordings of Adams's works, including the ten-CD collection of works published between the late 1970s and the
late 1990s titled *The John Adams Earbox*, released in 1999. Their linked webpage
devoted to Adams contains a biography of the composer, album releases for purchase, select compact-disc liner notes, tour information, upcoming conducting
engagements, and brief video interviews with Adams speaking on select works,
including *Short Ride in a Fast Machine*, *The Wound-Dresser*, Chamber Symphony,
Lollapalooza, *Hallelujah Junction*, *Road Movies*, *City Noir*, *Scheherazade.2*.

265.   *National Public Radio.* "John Adams." Accessed May 16, 2019. www.npr.org.

National Public Radio has hosted John Adams on numerous occasions. NPR
archives all their interviews and programs; among them include sessions with
Adams (or speaking about his musical works in his absence) on *Morning Edition*, *Weekend Edition*, *Deceptive Cadence*, *Fresh Air*, and *All Things Considered*.
Content on Adams can be searched from the homepage. NPR has also dedicated a webpage to Adams: www.npr.org/artists/14996733/john-adams. Also,
recording reviews and music articles pertaining to performances of his works
can be found.

The subjects explored in NPR provide invaluable insight into Adams's thoughts,
such as *The Death of Klinghoffer* and the controversies behind it, or the writing
of *On the Transmigration of Souls*, commissioned by the New York Philharmonic
in remembrance of September 11 victims. In a 2011 interview, Adams probes
further into his work *On the Transmigration of Souls*. Adams believed the audience should not relive the event with images, narrative reiteration, or dramatiza-
tion. The text stems from notes people posted around Ground Zero following the
attack. Adams opines that plain musical phrases with a simple language suited
the work. Adams turned to Ives as a model, with the rationale of preventing the
exploitation of emotions.

In a 2019 interview, Lloyd Schwartz talks with baritone Gerald Finley on his role as Robert Oppenheimer in the new recording of *Doctor Atomic* (www. npr.org/2019/01/14/685106876/new-recording-of-doctor-atomic-may-be-the-opera-s-definitive-performance).

In a 2015 live-recorded interview titled "John Adams Mines Beethoven's Mind," Adams discusses his own works inspired by Beethoven, including *Grand Pianola Music* and *Absolute Jest*. Adams relates that Stravinsky engaged in a similar process for composing *Pulcinella*. The interview compares music clips from Beethoven and Adams as he discusses his approach in more detail (www.npr. org/sections/deceptivecadence/2015/11/10/450560466/john-adams-mines-beethovens-mind). Another interview on this topic appears in 2012 with Michael Tilson Thomas, John Adams, and several other prominent musicians. Adams explains he derived his ideas using fragments from Beethoven's String Quartets Op. 131 and 135, and he fused the opening harmonic progression from his Piano Sonata No. 21 in C Major, Op. 53, known as the *Waldstein*.

A 2014 interview from *Deceptive Cadence* explores Adams's *The Gospel According to the Other Mary*. Adams touches upon sources for the libretto and its characters, and the role of women in the oratorio. Adams draws parallels on the treatment of the downtrodden to Mary Magdalene and present-day injustices (www.npr.org/sections/deceptivecadence/2014/03/23/292453186/john-adams-psychedelic-oratorio-gives-voice-to-the-other-mary).

In a 2013 interview, conductor David Robertson reflects on Adams's achievements in stamping a signature American sound for our time and examines the changing perception of symphonic writing during Adams's *Harmonielehre* and today (www.npr.org/sections/ deceptivecadence/2013/08/12/211376496/why-are-american-orchestras-afraid-of-new-symphonies).

266. *Opera News*. "John Adams." Accessed May 16, 2019. www.operanews.com.

Opera News features a number of articles about Adams's operas. Some of these articles highlight performers who participated in Adams's world premieres of works such as *The Gospel According to the Other Mary*. Other content includes recording reviews of *Doctor Atomic* and other works, collaborations with Peter Sellars, the Met's canceling of the live simulcast of *The Death of Klinghoffer*, and staging Adams's operas in the Théâtre du Châtelet 2013 in Paris. Opera News lists Adams as one of the twenty-five most powerful names in opera. Lastly, Opera News contains a 2009 interview with John Adams and Adam Wasserman on *A Flowering Tree*. This interview explores Adams's inspiration from an Indian folk tale and his aim to create a simple compositional style while embracing a multilingual perspective for this opera (www.operanews.com/operanews/issue/article.aspx?id=5018).

267. *PBS NewsHour*. "John Adams." Accessed May 16, 2019. www.pbs.org/newshour.

PBS NewsHour offers various video interviews with Adams. Journalist Jeffrey Brown interviews Adams in November 22, 2017 about his new opera

Girls of the Golden West. Adams and his collaborator and librettist Peter Sellars attempt to portray the realities of the California Gold Rush as told by minority groups from that period. Adams views their approach to storytelling as a more honest version of history that accounts for diverse points of view. This manner of plot creation and attempting to present a story without nationalistic biases is central to Adams's works. Adams objects to critics' opinions that he is a political composer, stating they have warped opinions about classical music using present-day topics (www.pbs.org/newshour/show/in-john-adams-new-gold-rush-opera-cultures-clash-with-a-tragic-ending).

In a 2014 video interview, Adams defends *The Death of Klinghoffer* amid attacks from prominent figures such as politician Rudy Giuliani and director of the Anti-Defamation League, Abraham Foxman. Adams speaks of artists' duty to raise human conflicts to another plane unmatched by history books (www.pbs.org/newshour/show/opera-depicting-modern-tragedy-sparks-protest).

10

Related Writings on Minimalism

268.   Avant-Rossi, Joan. "Michael Nyman: *The Man Who Mistook His Wife for a Hat.*" Master's thesis, University of North Texas, 2008.

Avant-Rossi examines Nyman's one-act chamber opera *The Man Who Mistook His Wife for a Hat*, written in 1986. She compares Nyman's musical style to that of Glass and Adams. The author notes that Adams's first opera, *Nixon in China*, employs minimalist techniques in a freer manner than Glass's *Einstein on the Beach*, notably in the presence of repetitive ascending scales, as well as its reiterated text and musical phrases from the chorus. The author draws other comparisons between Glass and Adams's operas in their libretti and their use of harmony. Adams favors a linear narrative corresponding with the events of the opera and greater use of chromaticism.

269.   Fink, Robert Wallace. *Repeating Ourselves: American Minimal Music as Cultural Practice*. Berkeley: University of California Press, 2005.

Fink provides a contrasting historical narrative for the genesis of minimalism, arguing that its origins reflect a post-World War II American society of consumers, mass media, and production. Most of Fink's commentary and analysis is devoted to the minimalist composer Steve Reich. Fink weaves Adams's thoughts on Baroque music in light of the "barococo" revival, noting that during Adams's early career, the composer was a "detractor" of minimalist and Baroque music, wishing to distance himself from "the silly chatter of baroque sequences and the stupefying repetitions of minimalist music" (173). Adams prefers to characterize himself as a composer who transcends the pervasive musical style of his time, as he believes J. S. Bach's music accomplished in the midst of the Baroque era.

270.   McClary, Susan. *Feminine Endings: Music, Gender, and Sexuality*. Minneapolis: University of Minnesota Press, 1991.

McClary gives a passing reference to Adams's *Harmonielehre* in a single paragraph and an extended footnote. Her approach to Adams, however peripheral in treatment, remains mostly uncharted in the study of his works. McClary subscribes to the notion that musical works like Adams's *Harmonielehre* are constructed from a narrative schema mirroring libidinal and sexual energy. McClary cites Adams's words from the linear notes of the first *Nonesuch* recording, where the composer uses imagery in terms of impotence and what she describes as "phallic explosions" (196).

271.   Struble, John Warthen. *The History of American Classical Music: MacDowell Through Minimalism*. New York: Facts on File, 1995.

Struble writes about the history of American music from MacDowell and the Second New England School to minimalism. The author devotes his attention to minimalism in the penultimate chapter, asserting the origins of the term stem from painting and sculpture. Struble brands La Monte Young as the founder of minimalism and then turns his attention to Terry Riley, Steve Reich, Philip Glass, and John Adams.

Struble mentions a handful of Adams's works in passing and without musical examples. Struble purports that Adams's approach to opera writing is more conservative than that of other minimalists, claiming to use conventional plot structures, together with traditional orchestra settings and vocal writing. His characterization of Adams's music is debatable; other scholars have argued that Adams, as the first postminimalist, steered the aesthetic into a freer and more intuitive compositional style. Disparaging reviews like Struble's were typical during the 1990s before Adams became one of the most widely acclaimed American composers.

11

Miscellaneous

272. Boss, Jack, Brad Osborn, Tim S. Pack, and Stephen Rodgers, eds. *Analyzing the Music of Living Composers (and Others)*. Newcastle upon Tyne: Cambridge Scholars, 2013.

Analyzing the Music of Living Composers (and Others) does not offer content on the music of John Adams; notwithstanding, the book contains two relevant chapters for the analysis of postminimalist works. In Chapter 1, Brent Yorgason explores musical processes in Michael Torke's *Telephone Book*. To situate the postminimalist timeframe, the author cites Timothy A. Johnson's 1994 article "Minimalism: Aesthetic, Style, or Technique" (see item 48). Yorgason enumerates specific conditions for a postminimalist style: speeding up musical processes, using musical processes in combination, and combining minimalist processes with other compositional techniques, be they cyclical patterns reminiscent of Stravinsky, motivic transformations in the style of Brahms, or the infusion of jazz elements. Yorgason describes Torke's musical process of static transposition, a compositional method of repeating musical patterns across a variety of keys—music theorists use the synonymous term *key-signature transformation*. In Chapter 3, Erik Heine offers an analysis of Arvo Pärt's *Arbos*. Closer inspection reveals Pärt utilized modal materials during the time Adams was composing his early gate works.

273. Bernard, Jonathan W. "Theory, Analysis, and the 'Problem' of Minimal Music." In *Concert Music, Rock and Jazz Since 1945: Essays and Analytical Studies*, eds. Elizabeth West Marvin and Richard Hermann, 259–84. Rochester: University of Rochester Press, 1995.

Bernard aims to capture the essence of minimalist music by ruling out some misconceptions: it is not static or non-Western, and it does not aim to hypnotize listeners. The music of Adams is mentioned only in passing, yet Bernard's analyses of Glass's *Music in Twelve Parts* and Reich's *Music for 18 Musicians* serve as models for understanding Adams's modular compositions and other early works.

274.   Buchler, Michael. "The Sonic Illusion of Metrical Consistency in Minimalist Composition." In *Proceedings of the 9th International Conference on Music Perception and Cognition*, eds. Mario Baroni, Anna Rita Addessi, Roberto Caterina, and Marco Costa, 697–701. Bologna: Bononga University Press, 2006.

Buchler provides a study of meter and rhythm in minimalist music, examining Adams's *Lollapalooza* as a case study. Buchler considers different philosophies of meter and rhythm by authors including Lerdahl and Jackendoff, Palmer and Krumhansl, Hasty, and Horlacher to ascertain the most appropriate approach for minimalist music. The author concludes that the more recent theories by Hasty and Horlacher are more appropriate for the analysis of Adams's music because they ascribe to a more causal relationship between meter and rhythm. Where Lerdahl and Jackendoff think of meter as a fixed property, Hasty asserts that rhythms can define meter. Taking this perspective, Buchler makes the case that repetitive patterns lead to metrical understanding. Buchler purports that in *Lollapalooza*, the opening bass ostinato forms the primary metrical layer. Shortly after, a competing repetitive pattern challenges a listener's perspective of meter through metrical dissonance. *Lollapalooza* oscillates between what is described as a grouping dissonance and a displacement dissonance, and according to the author, this stylistic trait diverges from Reich, Torke, or other minimalists. As Adams's work unfolds, Buchler points out how the sense of meter is further obscured by irregular iterations of each ostinato. The author believes that the small metrical deviations in Adams's *Lollapalooza* result in an illusory sense of metrical consistency.

275.   Cahill, Sarah. "Century Rolls (1996)." *Lincoln Center's John Adams Festival Program Book* (2003). Reprinted in *The John Adams Reader: Essential Writings on an American Composer*, ed. Thomas May, 160–2. Pompton Plains: Amadeus, 2006.

Cahill begins with a quotation of Adams describing his piano concerto *Century Rolls* as an attempt to recapture the feeling of listening to music recorded on piano rolls. Adams's words serve as a commentary on the effect of piano rolls on twentieth-century music composition, and *Century Rolls* is his response to what piano roll music might have sounded like today. Cahill discusses the influence of these piano rolls; one hears distant echoes (but not direct quotations) from Ravel's two concertos, Gershwin's Concerto in F, and Rachmaninoff's piano concerti. Even though the music is rooted in the present, Cahill states the concerto has some traditional aspects: the piano and orchestra parts are evenly matched, and the concerto consists of three movements. Cahill highlights noteworthy aspects of each movement. In the first movement, she calls attention to tonality and Adams's use of instrumentation. Regarding the second movement, which is cleverly titled "Manny's Gym," after the name of the dedicatee, pianist Emanuel Ax, Adams showcases a *gymnopédie* after Eric Satie, though it is not Adams's first use of this derivative form of composing—the first instance occurs in the "Aria of the Falling Body" in *The Death of Klinghoffer*. The third movement is well documented for its title typo "Hail Bop" based on the name of the 1995 comet Hale-Bopp. It is composed in a jazz style and conjures the feel of bebop and Jelly Roll Morton.

276.   ____. "Chamber Symphony (1992)." *Lincoln Center's John Adams Festival Program Book* (2003). Reprinted in *The John Adams Reader: Essential Writings on an American Composer*, ed. Thomas May, 149–50. Pompton Plains: Amadeus, 2006.

This article is all too brief to discuss Adams's Chamber Symphony in detail. Its readership was intended for concertgoers at the Lincoln Center's John Adams Festival. However, its brevity should not be confused for lack of content; indeed, Cahill brings up some important points in her program notes. First, Cahill purports that Chamber Symphony marks the beginning of a new compositional style for John Adams that is highly chromatic and polyphonic. Cahill draws attention to the now well-documented background of this work, having been influenced by an unusual mixture of Schoenberg's own *Kammersymphonie* and 1950s cartoon music. Then she notes differences between Adams and Schoenberg's chamber symphonies. Following a broad play-by-play of Adams's three movements, Cahill remarks additional sources for inspiration: Stravinsky's *L'Histoire du soldat*, Darius Milhaud's *La création du monde*, and Hindemith's *Kleine Kammermusik*.

277.   ____. "Grand Pianola Music (1982)." *Lincoln Center's John Adams Festival Program Book* (2003). Reprinted in *The John Adams Reader: Essential Writings on an American Composer*, ed. Thomas May, 89–90. Pompton Plains: Amadeus, 2006.

Cahill offers a succinct description of *Grand Pianola Music*, incorporating citations by the composer. She discusses Adams's phasing technique as stemming from the composer's own electronic experiments, rather than from Steve Reich's *Piano Phase* and other early minimalist works.

278.   ____. "*Fearful Symmetries* and *The Wound-Dresser* (1988)." Liner notes for *Fearful Symmetries/The Wound-Dresser* (1989 Nonesuch CD 7559-79218-2). Reprinted in *The John Adams Reader: Essential Writings on an American Composer*, ed. Thomas May, 120–6. Pompton Plains: Amadeus, 2006.

Cahill begins her notes with a quotation from Adams where he describes the experience of writing two divergent musical works during the same period— an abridged portion of Cahill's article appears in Adams's official website. *The Wound-Dresser*, representing Adams's darker and more serious personality, sets to music Walt Whitman's poem of the same title, scored for chamber orchestra and baritone, while *Fearful Symmetries*, a more rhythmically driven piece, explores Adams's more playful or "trickster" side. Cahill specifies what portions of Whitman's poem are excluded in Adams's musical depiction and offers a plausible explanation for the omission. Cahill's description of the pieces pays special attention to issues of orchestration; particularly how Adams's instrumentation transforms the mood of *The Wound Dresser* and the way instrumental colors and timbres achieve a sense of motion in *Fearful Symmetries*.

279.   Cott, Jonathan. "An Interview with John Adams by Jonathan Cott." *Harmonielehre*. Liner Notes for Nonesuch Digital 9 79115-2, 1985. Compact Disc.

This interview has been reprinted in Jonathan Cott's 2002 compilation *Back to a Shadow in the Night: Music Writings and Interviews, 1968–2001*. The interview provides an in-depth look at Adams's *Harmonielehre*. Adams experienced a dream of a tanker rising from the water near the Bay Bridge—this image propelled Adams's work. Adams explains he does not create a blueprint to a composition prior to embarking on a large work like *Harmonielehre*. This idea is in line with K. Robert Schwarz's assertion that Adams's style evolved from process-driven pieces using precomposed musical structures toward intuitive pieces whose structure takes shape as the piece unfolds. Adams dislikes describing his music as a continuous development of motivic material in a Germanic tradition. Instead, he prefers to think of his music akin to Sibelius's manner of creating musical continuity. In regards to the second movement, Adams ties in the darker affect, as it is a piece about physical and spiritual sickness. Adams portrays the working with keys in a similar fashion to the concept of ethos for the ancient Greeks, though Adams believes the emotional power in his music is achieved through an exploration of different tonalities and keys. Another interesting insight Adams offers is the work's polytonality, a technique that seems paradoxical for a composer who evaluates his musical style as tonal and consonant. Regarding the third movement, Adams claims he composed the opening measures using seven-voice counterpoint. If this claim is supported by his music, it presents an admirable feat of contrapuntal ingenuity, worthy of further investigation.

280.   Goodman, Alice. *History Is Our Mother: Three Libretti: Nixon in China, the Death of Klinghoffer, the Magic Flute*. New York: New York Review of Books, 2017.

Goodman compiles her libretti of *Nixon in China* and *The Death of Klinghoffer*, as well as her own English translation of *The Magic Flute* that she completed for a British production in 1991. Goodman's aim in this libretto compilation is to facilitate its study by focusing attention to all aspects of the prose, including form, rhythm, and lineation. Goodman gives detailed information on premiere performance dates and venues, production credits, and original cast members. The production credits include all facets of the opera production, ranging from music and libretto to director, conductor, choreographer, and costume, set, and lighting designers. Goodman's book also contains an introduction by James Williams, known for his scholarship on American literature.

As an interesting side note, Williams remarks that an unnamed opera-house director endorsed the well-known British novelist Doris Lessing as the librettist for the opera, though Sellars opted for his college friend Alice Goodman. Williams dispels any misconceptions about satire in *Nixon in China*; Goodman agreed to embark on this libretto with the condition that its theme would be that of a heroic opera. Williams offers an interpretation of various metaphors and allusions in Goodman's *Nixon in China*, most notably, "History is Our Mother." Williams ventures to explore the boundaries between history, politics, and mythology, drawing parallels to Beethoven's *Fidelio* as a like-minded opera in its treatment of recent history. In the latter part of his introduction, Williams describes Goodman's background as a writer and attempts to encapsulate her style. Williams describes Goodman's *The Death of Klinghoffer* as a libretto of juxtapositions, between biblical narrative and modern conflict, Jewish American vernacular and Palestinian disenfranchisement. Goodman's version of the libretto in this compilation is the original one that includes the controversial "Rumors" scene. Williams weighs in on the attack of the libretto as having anti-Semitic undertones, siding with Goodman and arguably giving the most detailed and persuasive published defense through his interpretation of the text.

281. Marshall, Ingram. "*Light Over Water*: The Genesis of a Music (1983)." *Available Light*, Los Angeles Museum of Contemporary Art (1983). Reprinted in *The John Adams Reader: Essential Writings on an American Composer*, ed. Thomas May, 91–100. Pompton Plains: Amadeus, 2006.

Little has been written about Adams's 1983 electronic work composed as a collaboration of music and dance with choreographer Lucinda Childs for the Los Angeles Museum of Contemporary Art. This essay first appeared in the 1985 LP recording New Albion 005. Marshall notes that *Light Over Water* is music for dance, and as such, it has a kind of subdued nature. Marshall describes the tripartite structure of the work in depth. Part I begins with an attacking sound in the synthesizer and low brasses, eventually quieting into "periodic rustlings of a dreaming sleeper" (96). Part II is composed in a binary form with a *pastorale* that leads into a "gently rolling continuum" (97). Part III employs dissonant polytonal modulations that increase the sense of motion. The remainder of the article includes quotations from Adams himself on the process of collaborating with Lucinda Childs.

282. ____. "*Naive and Sentimental Music*: A Sentimental Journey (1997–1998)." Liner notes from Nonesuch 7559-79636-2 compact disc (2002). Reprinted in *The John Adams Reader: Essential Writings on an American Composer*, ed. Thomas May, 163–70. Pompton Plains: Amadeus, 2006.

Ingram Marshall, fellow composer and friend of John Adams, wrote these liner notes on the 2002 Nonesuch record label. The title of Adams's work comes from the German poet Friedrich Schiller, but Marshall explains that it was Isaiah Berlin's 1968 essay "The Naiveté of Verdi" that formed Adams's thoughts on the matter. As is well known through Adams's writings, *Naive and Sentimental Music* is a symphony about artistic personalities: the naive are those "for whom art is a natural form of expression, uncompromised by self-analysis or worry over its place in the historical continuum," whereas the sentimental personality is self-aware (164).

As a musical depiction of naive versus sentimental, the author points to the opening movement played simply by the strumming of a guitar with a flute and oboe melody transcending over the accompaniment. However, in this description, it remains unclear when and how a passage ceases to be naive. According to Marshall, this symphony parallels Adams's development as a composer, initially writing works influenced by the early minimalists, who were naive in their conception of a budding musical style. Yet Adams's works succeeding *Nixon in China* take a more sentimental, intellectually self-aware form. The second movement, titled "Mother of the Man," is a heartfelt commentary on Ferruccio Busoni's *Berceuse élégiaque*. Marshall makes an interesting connection between this style of *gymnopédie* writing and others from Adams's oeuvre: the "Aria of the Falling Body" from *The Death of Klinghoffer*; the "Manny's Gym" movement from *Century Rolls*, and the chaconne from the Violin Concerto. These pieces are "dreamlike, almost motionless, cyclical essays in suspended animation" (167). On a final note, Marshall believes that Adams's *Naive and Sentimental Music* is written in a landscape genre akin to *El Dorado*.

283.   ____. "Shaker Loops (1978; revised 1983)." *San Francisco Symphony Program Book* (September 1983). Reprinted in *The John Adams Reader: Essential Writings on an American Composer*, ed. Thomas May, 74–9. Pompton Plains: Amadeus, 2006.

Fellow composer Ingram Marshall discusses the creation and evolution of *Shaker Loops* from its chamber string format, derived out of a work called *Wavemaker*, to the 1983 revised version for string orchestra. Marshal explains that Adams was dissatisfied with the 1978 chamber string version and withdrew it from performance. The early version of *Shaker Loops* was written using modules that give the conductor control over timing and placement of entrances. For practical purposes, the 1983 version is written out in a manner that Adams found most successful. Marshall details the origin of the title and gives a broad analysis of each of the four movements. Marshall employs a tonal style of analysis, identifying key structures and diatonic modes evidenced in the score. This is consistent with Adams's early style of writing in other pieces such as *Phrygian Gates*.

284.   Mertens, Wim. *American Minimal Music: La Monte Young, Terry Riley, Steve Reich, Philip Glass*. Translated by Jan Hautekiet. London: Kahn & Averill, 1983.

Mertens's book presents a good introduction to early minimalist music. The author devotes individual chapters to the four founders of minimalism, though he omits discussion of Adams and postminimalist works. Nevertheless, readers become acquainted with Mertens's perspective on the historical development of minimalism, along with basic concepts, and invaluable information on musical movements leading up to American minimalism. Mertens engages with writings by Adorno to offer a unique viewpoint of minimalism, stating that Adorno's confrontation with the progress of music and time has been thwarted by minimalist composers. He also entertains the Freudian notions from detractors of the minimalist aesthetic to consider whether repetitive music can lead to psychological regression.

285. "A Nonesuch Celebration." *Brooklyn Academy of Music, BAM Howard Gilman Opera House* (April 1, 2017). Accessed January 26, 2019. www.bam.org/media/9013184/Nonesuch.pdf.

Adams arranged a tribute to Robert Hurwitz, who was the president of Nonesuch Records from 1984 to 2017. John Adams asked a wide array of composers and songwriters who had worked with Hurwitz over the years at Nonesuch to compose a piece for him, to which every musician replied favorably. The culmination of these compositions resulted in a two-and-a-half-hour concert at the BAM Howard Gilman Opera House on April 1, 2017. The program included online contains a "Who's Who" that encompasses all the performers and composers who took part in this event. For the occasion, Adams composed his latest piano piece, *I Still Play*, written in a style that an inspired music amateur such as Hurwitz might play.

286. "Performance Studies: John Adams Topic Exploration Pack." *Oxford Cambridge and RSA Examinations* (September 2015). Accessed May 17, 2016. www.ocr.org.uk/Images/260978-john-adams-topic-exploration-pack.pdf.

Oxford Cambridge and RSA developed a number of teacher resource packs for study and examination purposes. The pack aids in the study of structure and form, elements of performing arts, performance techniques, and stylistic influences, as well as cultural, historical, and social context. The study guide is written in bullet points in an attempt to encapsulate Adams's musical style in a concise manner. One section of the guide is devoted to musical influences that shaped John Adams—it encompasses a wide range including John Cage, Steve Reich, jazz, electronics, rock music, romanticism, and Schoenberg. The second half of the guide strives to impart students with an understanding of Adams's early minimal style through the study of *Phrygian Gates*. Two interpretations of the musical structure of *Phrygian Gates* are presented, one as containing three movements and one that breaks the first section into two, thereby resulting in a four-movement work. Brief notes on musical parameters such as harmony, rhythm and meter, melody, and texture are explored. The last section of the guide outlines teaching lessons on the study of Adams's early piano work *Phrygian Gates*.

287. Ramaut-Chevassus, Béatrice. "L'énergie 'tonale': l'opéra selon John Adams." In *Des Ponts vers l'Amérique:* Proceedings of the CRAL/EHESS (*Centre de Recherces sur les Arts et le Langage*, and École des Hautes Études en Sciences Sociales), Paris, December 7–8, 2006. In French.

Ramaut-Chevassus writes on relations between American and European contemporary art music, focusing on Adams. She remarks that European composers view American composers with joint admiration and contempt. The author finds links between Adams and Europe, pointing to the production and world premieres of *The Death of Klinghoffer* in Brussels, *El Niño* in Paris, and *A Flowering Tree* in Vienna. In the course of her study, Ramaut-Chevassus alludes to her argument: if Adams's operatic works reject the foundational principles of

American modernist movements such as Cageian indeterminacy and early minimalist techniques in lieu of a dramatic and eclectic style of minimalism, then his approach corresponds more closely to a cosmopolitan style that bridges European and American musical traditions.

288.   Roeder, John. "Beat-Class Modulation in Steve Reich's Music." *Music Theory Spectrum* 25, no. 2 (2003): 275–304.

Roeder develops a rhythmic model for the analysis of textural form in Reich's recent works. Theoretical studies on rhythm and meter in minimalist music are scant, and while Roeder's article is devoted strictly to Reich, his models are easily transferrable to Adams's earlier minimalist works, including *Shaker Loops* and *Lollapalooza*, to name a few.

289.   ____. "Transformational Aspects of Arvo Pärt's Tintinnabuli Music." *Journal of Music Theory* 55, no. 1 (2011): 1–41.

Roeder applies transformational analysis—influenced by David Lewin's seminal 1987 *Generalized Musical Intervals and Transformations*—and neo-Riemannian theoretical tools to examine Pärt's procedure for creating harmonic constructs called *tintinnabulation*. Adams is not referenced in Roeder's study, yet his analytical tools could supplement studies on Adams's works that employ a neo-Riemannian approach.

290.   Schwarz, K. Robert. "Remaking American Opera." *Institute for Studies in American Music Newsletter* 24, no. 2 (1995): 1–2, 14–15.

Schwarz's article offers snippets from an interview he facilitated with the composers John Adams, Anthony Davis, Meredith Monk, and Tania León in 1994 at the City University of New York Graduate Center. The interview delves into the genre of contemporary opera writing. Adams recounts his first experience with opera, going to the Met to hear Verdi's *Aida* when he was a junior in high school and recalling he did not care for the experience. Adams candidly admits not being an opera aficionado prior to embarking on a compositional career of writing operas himself.

291.   Sirota, Nadia. "Splitting Adams: John Adams' Chamber Symphonies" (April 19, 2017). Accessed April 7, 2019. www.newsounds.org/story/splitting-adams-john-adams-chamber-symphonies.

Violist Nadia Sirota and conductor Alan Pierson of the chamber ensemble *Alarm Will Sound* provide part interview with Adams and part podcast on the subject of his two chamber symphonies. Adams composed *Son of Chamber Symphony* for this ensemble, who premiered the work in 2007. Sirota and Pierson elaborate on performance aspects of both chamber symphonies. The performers give a recollection of their rehearsal with Adams, speaking on performance challenges, issues of balancing instruments, and the composer's small revisions upon hearing his music performed. Sirota remarks that Adams would make revisions to suit the performers' strengths, and in this sense, Adams's compositions entail a collaboration between composer and performers. Adams speaks on the background of a few of his titles from his oeuvre, including *Son of Chamber Symphony*. Sirota and Pierson touch upon other interesting aspects of Adams's chamber work, including Adams's short motivic idea that is reminiscent of Beethoven's Symphony No. 9, and his return to his minimalist roots, most notably in the last movement.

292.   Sontag, Susan. "A Lexicon for *Available Light*." *Art in America* 71 (1983): 100–10. Reprinted in *Where the Stress Falls: Essays*, 161–77. New York: Farrar, Straus, and Giroux, 2001.

Sontag analyzes the dance work *Available Light*, a collaboration between John Adams, choreographer Lucinda Childs, and architect Frank Gehry. Adams subsequently recorded his music for *Available Light* under the name *Light Over Water*. While Sontag does not provide a direct discussion of Adams's music, her lexicon gives a rare overview of *Available Light*. The author presents an extensive list of topics on their collaboration: beauty, choreography, complexity, Cunningham, dance, diagonal, doubling, *Einstein on the Beach*, emotion, formations, geometrical, head, ideal, illustrating, Judson Dance Theater, Kleist's Essay on the Puppet Theatre, lightness, measurable, minimalist, movements, neo-classical, openings, order, politeness, post-modern, presence/absence, quartets, *Relative Calm*, repetition, romantic, solos, space, titles, unavailable, volition, world, yearning, and *Zeno's Territory*. Sontag elaborates on signature elements of Childs's choreography (diagonal, doubling, formations) and explains that Childs ascribed to the philosophy that dance should not express references to emotions, stories, or landscapes.

293.   Steinberg, Michael. "*The Death of Klinghoffer* (1990–91)." Liner notes for *The Death of Klinghoffer*, Nonesuch 7559-79281-2 (1992). Reprinted in *The John Adams Reader: Essential Writings on an American Composer*, ed. Thomas May, 127–42. Pompton Plains: Amadeus, 2006.

Steinberg compares and contrasts Adams's first two operas. Some similarities are transparent, such as the Adams-Goodman-Sellars trio working together, or the return of cast members from their first opera, or the subject matter stemming from relatively current events. That is where the similarities end, claims Steinberg. He reaffirms Adams and Sellars's point that their work seeks inspiration from Bach's *Passions* for their complex layering of narrative and commentary. Steinberg includes a synopsis of the libretto, along with musical and analytical commentary to connect music and text.

294.   ____. "El Dorado." *San Francisco Symphony Program Book* (November 1991). Reprinted in *The John Adams Reader: Essential Writings on an American Composer*, ed. Thomas May, 143–8. Pompton Plains: Amadeus, 2006.

Steinberg begins this article by contextualizing *El Dorado* as an authentic 1990s work of art that expresses dissent towards the 80s decade for its greed and self-absorbed attitude. The name of the work is inspired by the tale of *El Dorado* that drew Spanish conquistadors to search for the lost city in vain. The first movement, originally titled "Pizarro's Dream" and subsequently changed to "A Dream of Gold," is a reflection of humanity and its role in abusing the natural order. It is interesting that Adams musically captures this sentiment by employing the minimalist style, yet in an atonal fashion. Steinberg explains how *El Dorado* shares a connection to *Harmonielehre*: both works are directly influenced by the composer Sibelius, but whereas *Harmonielehre* draws from the Fourth Symphony, *El Dorado* emulates the harmonic language of Sibelius's Sixth Symphony. The second movement, titled "Soledades," portrays *El Dorado* without the influence of man. Musically, Adams creates this effect with tonal-sounding minimalist harmonies. Steinberg includes a broad analysis of both movements. The first movement contains chromaticism and the presence of the octatonic scale. The second movement resides in a modal world akin to Sibelius's Symphony. A connection not discussed by Steinberg entails the second movement of *El Dorado* and the first movement of *Naive and Sentimental Music*, where Adams conceives a parallel treatment of harmony, orchestration, and instrumentation.

295.   ____. "El Niño: A Nativity Oratorio (1999–2000)." Liner notes for El Niño, Nonesuch, 2002. Reprinted in *The John Adams Reader: Essential Writings on an American Composer*, ed. Thomas May, 171–82. Pompton Plains: Amadeus, 2006.

El Niño—initially titled *How Could This Happen*, after a phrase in a motet by the composer Orlande de Lassus—is a musical work that can be performed as a staged production or as a concert oratorio. Steinberg explains the text comes from a wide variety of sources in Spanish, Latin, and English, including poems by Rosario Castellanos, Gabriela Mistral, Hildegard von Bingen, Sor Juana Inés de la Cruz, Rubén Darío, and Vicente Huidobro, and passages from the Bible, the New Testament Apocrypha, and The Wakefield Mystery Plays. The work was dedicated to Adams's longtime collaborator Peter Sellars, who directed the first production and shaped the work in its entirety. Steinberg summarizes how a commission from the San Francisco Symphony and the Paris Théâtre du Châtelet for an orchestra and chorus work resulted in Adams's oratorio.

The writing of *El Niño* was a voyage of self-discovery for Adams. He regards Handel's *Messiah* highly, and the composer admits having a desire to write his own *Messiah* as a way to understand his "checkered religious background" and look into his own psyche (173). Steinberg tells readers that *El Niño* is similar to Handel's *Messiah* in its "simplicity and directedness with which the words convey their message of belief, and in the joy the composer takes in setting English words to music" (175). Yet, unlike Handel, Adams wanted to bring focus on the nativity as the miracle of birth. For this reason, women's voices are at the forefront of the work.

Steinberg's liner notes include a meticulous synopsis of the oratorio, detailing poets and their texts and contextualizing their writing with Adams's musical settings. Steinberg references the opening of the oratorio as bearing some resemblance to Beethoven's Ninth Symphony for its effect and tonality, as well as *Harmonium*, for the repetition of a single syllable for an extended period. I wish Steinberg's writing would have engaged the reader with a discussion of the modal style of music (with a contemporary twist) that so prominently drives the arias and duets throughout the oratorio. Peter Sellars brings up this point in a 2006 interview with Thomas May, available in *The John Adams Reader*.

296.   ____. "*Harmonielehre* (1984–1985)." *San Francisco Symphony Program Book* (March 1985). Reprinted in *The John Adams Reader: Essential Writings on an American Composer*, ed. Thomas May, 101–5. Pompton Plains: Amadeus, 2006.

Steinberg writes an interesting account of how Adams conceived the idea for composing *Harmonielehre*. Adams struggled to write the large orchestral work for some time, though one night he dreamt he saw himself driving across the Bay Bridge looking out at a huge tanker, which suddenly took off like a rocket. This image gave Adams the impetus for his newest work; the next morning he worked out the opening measures of the opening movement. Adams offers more detail to the story on his official website. As Adams was putting finishing touches on *Harmonielehre*, he related to Steinberg the inspiration for his second movement came from Sibelius's Fourth Symphony. Another source for ideas was clearly Schoenberg for writing his well-known treatise on harmony. Steinberg introduces each movement from *Harmonielehre* in qualitative terms. The first movement features changing metrical patterns that are succeeded by slower music full of yearning. Of the second movement, Steinberg states Adams's harmonies revolve like an agonizingly slow kaleidoscope.

297.   ____. "*Harmonium* for Large Orchestra and Chorus (1980–1981)." *San Francisco Symphony Program Book* (April 1981). Reprinted in *The John Adams Reader: Essential Writings on an American Composer*, ed. Thomas May, 80–8. Pompton Plains: Amadeus, 2006.

This entry includes Steinberg's program notes from April 1981 and a chapter on *Harmonium* from his 2005 book *Choral Masterworks: A Listener's Guide* (its relevant section is found on pages 9–15). Steinberg, who was serving as artistic adviser for the San Francisco Symphony, reflects on the premiere of Adams's *Harmonium* performed in April 1981 at the Davies Hall in San Francisco. The program notes introduce John Adams to audiences largely unfamiliar with the up-and-coming composer. Steinberg examines the stylistic differences in Adams's choice of text from John Donne's "Negative Love" and Emily Dickinson's "Because I Could Not Stop for Death" and "Wild Nights." Adams's musical take for "Negative Love" begins with its well-known preamble consisting of iterations of the monosyllabic word "no" for several minutes, which later unfolds with Donne's first lines. Steinberg cites much of his information from an essay John Adams wrote in 1984 on *Harmonium*.

298.   ____. "*My Father Knew Charles Ives* (2003)." *San Francisco Symphony Program Book* (April 2003). Reprinted in *The John Adams Reader: Essential Writings on an American Composer*, ed. Thomas May, 205–8. Pompton Plains: Amadeus, 2006.

Steinberg purports that *My Father Knew Charles Ives* continues the musical-biographical genre originating with Berlioz's *Symphonie fantastique*. Steinberg notes that Adams believes there are similarities between the two composers and their relationship with their fathers. Adams's work is directly influenced by Ives's *Three Places in New England*; the composer writes three movements portraying three other places not depicted in Ives's work. The first movement, titled "Concord," refers to a small town in New Hampshire where Adams's parents grew up. It quotes reveille and a Beethoven duet for clarinet and bassoon Adams remembers playing as a boy. The method of layering textures in this movement is noteworthy. According to Steinberg, Adams translates geographical distances into musical layers using contrasting harmonic languages. The foreground layer is mostly tonal, the middle-ground layer is "ambivalently tonal," and the background is a less methodical, *pianissimo* texture (207). The second movement, titled "The Lake," refers to Lake Winnipesaukee, where Adams's parents met in a dance hall owned by his mother's stepfather. Here the evocation of jazz he used to hear as a boy is perceptible. The final movement, "The Mountain," written in a more contemplative affective quality, is more about Adams's relationship with the mountains behind his family house in Concord, but also with the West Coast and with nature as a whole.

299.   _____. *"Nixon in China* (1985–1987)." *Liner Notes for Nixon in China*, Nonesuch 7559-79177-2 (1988). Reprinted in *The John Adams Reader*, ed. Thomas May, 110–19. Pompton Plains: Amadeus, 2006.

Steinberg writes an excellent introduction to *Nixon in China*. The author situates Adams's opera within the opera tradition, drawing parallels from Wagner's *The Nibelung's Ring* (the meeting between Wotan and Erda being similar in magnitude to that between Nixon and Mao Tse-tung), as well as between Henry Kissinger, as an ominous figure in the opera, and *Tristan und Isolde*'s Melot, Tristan's seemingly loyal friend who betrays him. Steinberg includes abridged portions of Alice Goodman's libretto along with commentary and contextualizes various scenes of the opera to Adams's earlier works, such as *Harmonielehre*, where the author claims it was in this piece where Adams first gave "free reign to his lyric bent," now transforming that emotion-driven attribute to Pat Nixon's aria "This is prophetic" (117). The main point to be drawn from Steinberg's introduction is that *Nixon in China* is far more than a political opera; to characterize it as such detracts from all its complexities that make use of "the full potential of our cognitive resources" (113).

300.   _____. "Violin Concerto (1993)." *San Francisco Symphony Program Book* (January 2000). Reprinted in *The John Adams Reader*, ed. Thomas May, 151–7. Pompton Plains: Amadeus, 2006.

Steinberg furnishes much detail about the genesis of Adams's Violin Concerto. Steinberg writes about how Jorja Fleezanis, associate concertmaster of the San Francisco Symphony, first heard *Harmonielehre* on the radio in 1985 and was so thrilled with the piece she asked Adams to compose a violin concerto. The project took eight years to come to fruition because Fleezanis moved to Minnesota. Adams, not a violinist, found the project daunting but also exciting. So many composers before him have written some of the hallmarks of classical music through the medium of the violin concerto. Steinberg believes that Adams's Chamber Symphony was a kind of proving ground for Adams to test his abilities for string writing. Steinberg's article is the only one I have discovered that explains how Adams was able to remedy some of the challenges in writing for the violin. At first, he began using a T-square, a device invented by Donald Martino to learn what chords (multiple stops) are possible on the violin. Gradually, Adams began to trust his abilities more and consult with Fleezanis on writing for violin in a natural and idiomatic way. During the initial stages of writing the concerto, Adams conceived the work in two movements. Eventually, it transformed into a three-movement work. Steinberg details much information about each movement in light of other musical influences. In the second movement, for example, the author discusses Adams's *Chaconne* in contrast to chaconne and passacaglia bass lines found in Baroque music. Steinberg, in passing, also mentions how Adams made use of computer software in composing, though he does not probe further.

301. Warburton, Dan. "A Working Terminology for Minimal Music." *Intégral* 2 (1988): 135–59.

Warburton charts signature techniques of the minimalist style. The author targets Schenkerian analysis and pitch-class set theory as unsuitable models for understanding minimalist works. Warburton's attack on formalist models applies more directly to early minimalist works, as recent authors have devised elegant prolongational and set-class models to describe Adams's postminimalist style. Warburton's classification of minimalist techniques includes phasing, overlapping pattern work, dovetailing, and linear-, block-, and textural-additive processes. Several musical passages are included for illustration, though none by Adams.

302. Wiprud, Theodore and Joyce Lawler, eds. *Composer in Residence: Meet the Composer's Orchestra Residencies Program, 1982–1992.* Copyright 1995, Meet the Composer.

The *Composer in Residence* booklet, compiled by Wiprud and Lawler, provides information on John Adams's 1982–1985 residence with the San Francisco Symphony. During his residency, Adams composed and premiered *Harmonielehre* and revised *Christian Zeal and Activity* and *Common Tones in Simple Time*. The program funded Adams for a period of three years and bridged his transition from a part-time composer and college professor to a full-time composer—his $40,000 yearly grant was almost twice his salary as a college professor at the time. The support from this program was not only financial; it provided a network of composers, orchestras, performances, and recording opportunities that boosted his career to an international platform. Adams's official residency commission was *Harmonielehre*, and thanks in part to the residency, Adams was able to release a recording on a commercial label (Elektra/Nonesuch 79115-2, 1985) and give numerous performances of the work.

12

Encyclopedia Entries

303. Cahill, Sarah. "Adams, John (Coolidge)." In *Grove Music Online*, ed. Deane Root. Accessed September 20, 2016. http://www.oxfordmusiconline.com/subscriber/article/grove/music/42479.

Sarah Cahill's article offers an invaluable point of entry into John Adams's life, professional career, and compositional works. Cahill, who is a proponent of new music as a concert pianist and writer alike, is also a friend of the composer. Adams's first mature work for solo piano, titled *China Gates*, was dedicated to Cahill. In my correspondence with Cahill, the writer asserts that Adams approved the article's accuracy and content. Cahill's most recent update of her Grove Music entry appeared in 2008.

304. Fink, Robert. "(Post-)minimalisms 1970–2000: The Search for a New Mainstream." In *The Cambridge History of Twentieth-Century Music*, eds. Nicholas Cook and Anthony Pople, 539–56. Cambridge: Cambridge University Press, 2004.

Fink discusses the historical significance of minimalism, elaborating on different historical narratives, including Leonard Meyer's belief that aleatoric music would bring about a collapse of a four-hundred-year musical tradition that emanated from the Renaissance. Yet Fink presents a different narrative from Meyer, one that identifies the period between 1974 and 1982 as the culmination of pulse-patterned minimalism. Fink remarks that postminimalism was born under the shadow of minimalism and concurs with Timothy A. Johnson that its "new hospitality to traditional notions of craft and compositional voice now made it an attractive *stylistic* choice" (542). Fink demonstrates how

European modernist composers were drawn to the minimalist aesthetic. After expository prose on the minimalist style, Fink directs his attention to Adams's earlier works, purporting that Bryars was a probable influence on *Christian Zeal and Activity* and McGuire's *Variations* on *Phrygian Gates*. Fink places more importance on Adams's *Grand Pianola Music* than other scholars and marks it as the watershed moment when Adams broke free of earlier minimalist rigidity. According to Fink, minimalism achieved rising popularity in the 1980s and works such as Adams's *Harmonielehre* helped institutionalize the movement for widespread approval across American universities. Lastly, Fink devotes attention to Adams's first two operas and *El Niño* in his section entitled "Postminimalist Music Theater."

305. Taruskin, Richard. "A Harmonious Avant-Garde?" In *The Oxford History of Western Music*. Vol. 5. New York: Oxford University Press, 2005.

The fifth volume from Taruskin's *The Oxford History of Western Music* investigates the musical period following World War II. The author devotes his chapter "A Harmonious Avant-Garde?" to minimalist music. Taruskin notes how *Nixon in China* sprung a new wave of opera commissions during the 1990s. Taruskin describes Adams's postminimalist opera style as having "freely grouped and regrouped subtactile pulses and arpeggios of minimalism, and interesting textures obtained by pitting pulses at differing rates of speed in counterpoint, [which] were reconciled with a fairly conventional harmonic idiom, naturalistic vocal declamation, a neat 'numbers' format replete with entertaining choral and dance sequences, and frequent references to styles of popular music" (518). Taruskin asserts that Adams's harmonic language revolves around circles of major and minor thirds in place of the nineteenth-century harmonic practice of the circle of fifths. Taruskin contrasts Adams's polyharmonies to Stravinsky's Petrushka chord, yet its minimalist context unfolds in a seemingly consonant manner. Another harmonic feature Taruskin notes is the use of second-inversion triads, to which the composer "grants full rights of citizenship" (519).

Thinking about Adams's operas historically, Taruskin posits that *Nixon in China* diverges from disillusioned, post-World War I operas of the 1920s and 1930s by invoking opera's power of enchantment that turned Adams's political figures into godlike creatures. Taruskin proceeds to *The Death of Klinghoffer*, bringing up the same objections he has expressed in other earlier writings and stating that the transcendence of operatic characters into mythical figures is simply an arrogant evasion of moral judgment. Yet, despite Taruskin's condemnation of *Klinghoffer*, Adams enjoys international recognition due in part to the controversy of his opera.

The final section of Taruskin's take on music history summarizes what he sees as a trend in recent compositions toward sacred themes. One of the works under discussion is John Adams's *El Niño*. The author relates Adams's melodic idiom—in its application of large disjunct motion through wide intervals—to expressionism, relating one scene that depicts war and human slaughter. Similarly to his other reviews of Adams's works with text or a libretto, Taruskin critiques *El Niño* on grounds that audiences who are "looking for purifying experiences are easily beguiled by symbols of innocence" such as what the story of Adams's opera portrays (526). Furthermore, the author makes his opinion clear that Adams's depiction of the nativity is intended for unsophisticated audiences.

A

Discography of Adams's Compositions and Arrangements

Adams's works are organized alphabetically by title in this discography. The recordings for each composition appear in the order in which they were released. The discography includes the appropriate record label name and number, soloists, performing ensemble, and conductor. Other relevant information—such as dates and locations of recordings, timings, and production credits—can be accessed using online databases, most notably www.discogs.com, but also www.worldcat.org, www.discogs.com, www.boosey.com, and other resources from the San Francisco Symphony, Los Angeles Philharmonic, and others. I have made effort to include all readily available recordings to date, excluding re-released duplications of the same recordings, video recordings of Adams's operatic works, and a small number of compact discs that only feature one or several movements from a larger work. Most of the recordings available today are in compact disc format, although some older recordings are found in LP format and some newer ones on MP3 format, available online.

Two noteworthy recording compilations of Adams's works are available to music fans. The first is a ten-CD retrospective of Adams's works, titled *The John Adams Earbox*, released on the Nonesuch (79453-2) label in 1999. The contents of this collection include the following:

Chamber Symphony

Christian Zeal and Activity

Common Tones in Simple Time

El Dorado

Eros Piano

Fearful Symmetries

Five Songs

Gnarly Buttons

Grand Pianola Music

Harmonielehre

Harmonium

Hoodoo Zephyr

I Was Looking at the Ceiling and Then I Saw the Sky

John's Books of Alleged Dances

Lollapalooza

Nixon in China

Shaker Loops

Slonimsky's Earbox

The Chairman Dances

The Death of Klinghoffer

The Wound-Dresser

Two Fanfares for Orchestra

Violin Concerto

All of the selections in this ten-disc collection have been previously released on Nonesuch, except for Harmonium, Lollapalooza, and Slonimsky's Earbox, which are detailed individually in this discography. These three works were subsequently released individually in 2000 in Nonesuch 7559-79549-2 and Nonesuch 7559-79607-2.

The second compilation of Adams's works was released in 2017 by the Berliner Philharmoniker Recordings (BPHR 17041) label. This collection contains four CDs and two Blu-ray discs featuring the following musical works and additional content:

City Noir

Harmonielehre

Lollapalooza

Scheherazade.2

Short Ride in a Fast Machine

The Gospel According to the Other Mary

The Wound-DresserConcert Recordings in High Definition Video

John Adams in Conversation with Sarah Willis

John Adams in Conversation with Peter Sellars

A Portrait of John Adams as the Berliner Philharmoniker's Composer in Residence

A FLOWERING TREE

Nonesuch 327100-2 (CD) (2008)

Soloists: Jessica Rivera, soprano; Russel Thomas, tenor; Eric Owens, bass-baritone

Ensembles: London Symphony Orchestra; Schola Cantorum de Venezuela

Conductor: John Adams

ABSOLUTE JEST

SFS Media 0063 (CD) (2015)

Ensembles: St. Lawrence String Quartet; San Francisco Symphony

Conductor: Michael Tilson Thomas

Chandos 5199 (CD) (2018)

Ensembles: Doric String Quartet; Royal Scottish National Orchestra

Conductor: Peter Oundjian

AMERICAN BERSERK

Nonesuch 7559796992 (CD) (2004)

Soloist: Nicolas Hodges, piano

Naxos American Classics 8.559285 (CD) (2007)

Soloist: Ralph van Raat, piano

Brilliant Classics 95388 (CD) (2017)

Soloist: Jeroen van Veen

Skulpturenpark Waldfrieden CF 003 (CD) (2017)

Soloist: Holger Groschopp

AMERICAN STANDARD

Obscure Records 2-A (LP) (1975)

Ensemble: The New Music Ensemble of the San Francisco Conservatory of Music

Other information: Produced by Brian Eno

BERCEUSE ÉLÉGIAQUE (ARRANGEMENT)

Nonesuch 7559-79359-2 (CD) (1996)
Ensemble: London Sinfonietta
Conductor: John Adams

Naxos 8.559031 (CD) (2004)
Ensemble: Bournemouth Symphony Orchestra
Conductor: Marin Alsop

Jupiter Records 109 (CD) (2007)
Ensemble: London Symphony Orchestra
Conductor: Gisèle Ben-Dor

CENTURY ROLLS

Nonesuch 7559-79607-2 (CD) (2000)
Soloist: Emanuel Ax, piano
Ensemble: The Cleveland Orchestra
Conductor: Christoph von Dohnanyi

Prior Records 043/044 (CD) (2010)
Soloist: Petras Geniušas
Ensemble: Lithuanian National Symphony Orchestra
Conductor: Juozas Domarkas

CHAMBER SYMPHONY

Nonesuch 7559-79219-2 (CD) (1994)
Ensemble: London Sinfonietta
Conductor: John Adams

RCA Victor Red Seal 09026-68674-2 (CD) (1997)
Ensemble: Ensemble Modern
Conductor: Sian Edwards

Actes Sud 34102 (CD) (1999)

Ensemble: Orchestre Philharmonique de Montpellier L.-R.

Conductor: René Bosc

CCn'C Records 492 (CD) (1999)

Ensemble: Absolute Ensemble

Conductor: Kristjan Järvi

Etcetera Records KTC 9000 (CD) (2006)

Ensemble: Schönberg Ensemble

Conductor: Reinbert de Leeuw

Cantaloupe Music CA21128 (CD) (2017)

Ensemble: Alarm Will Sound

Conductor: Alan Pierson

CHINA GATES

Argo 436 925 (CD) (1993)

Soloist: Alan Feinberg

TROY 038 (CD) (1993)

Soloist: Christopher O'Riley

Tall Poppies 108 (CD) (1997)

Soloist: Peter Waters

Pianovox 510 (CD) (1998)

Soloist: Jay Gottlieb

Telarc 80513 (CD) (1998)

Soloist: Gloria Cheng-Cochran

BIS Records 1110 (CD) (2000)

Soloist: Jenny Lin

Stradivarius 33555 (CD) (2000)

Soloist: Emanuele Arciuli

Arabesque Recordings 6776 (CD) (2003)
Soloist: Bruce Brubaker

Nonesuch 7559796992 (CD) (2004)
Soloist: Nicolas Hodges

Black Box Classics 1098 (CD) (2005)
Soloist: Andrew Russo

Brilliant Classics 8551 (CD) (2007)
Soloist: Jeroen van Veen

Naxos American Classics 8.559285 (CD) (2007)
Soloist: Ralph van Raat

Yarlung Records 79580 (CD) (2008)
Soloist: Joanne Pearce Martin

Roger McVey 884501173476 (MP3) (2009)
Soloist: Roger McVey

ATMA Classique 22556 (CD) (2010)
Soloist: David Jalbert

Con Brio Recordings 21046 (CD) (2011)
Soloist: Jocelyn Swigger

Fleur de Son 58006 (CD) (2012)
Soloist: John Milbauer

TROY 1342 (CD) (2012)
Soloist: Molly Morkoski

Canary Classics 11 (CD) (2014)
Soloist: Orli Shaham

Helisek Music Publishing 0239 (CD) (2014)
Soloist: Timothy A. Helisek

Mirare 239 (CD) (2014)
Soloist: Shani Diluka

KAIROS 13292 (CD) (2015)
Soloist: Marino Formenti

TROY 1617 (CD) (2016)
Soloist: Sung-Soo Cho

Brilliant Classics 95388 (CD) (2017)
Soloist: Jeroen van Veen

Skulpturenpark Waldfrieden CF 003 (CD) (2017)
Soloist: Holger Groschopp

Zefir Records 9654 (CD) (2018)
Soloist: Feico Deutekom

CHRISTIAN ZEAL AND ACTIVITY

Obscure Records 2-A (LP) (1975)
Ensemble: The New Music Ensemble of the San Francisco Conservatory of Music
Other information: Produced by Brian Eno

Nonesuch 7559-79144-2 (CD) (1987)
Ensemble: San Francisco Symphony
Conductor: Edo de Waart

Actes Sud 34102 (CD) (1999)
Ensemble: Orchestre Philharmonique de Montpellier L.-R.
Conductor: René Bosc

CITY NOIR

Nonesuch 7559-79564-4 (CD) (2014)
Ensemble: Saint Louis Symphony Orchestra
Conductor: David Robertson

COMMON TONES IN SIMPLE TIME

Nonesuch 7559-79144-2 (CD) (1987)

Ensemble: San Francisco Symphony

Conductor: Edo de Waart

DOCTOR ATOMIC

Nonesuch 7559-79310-7 (CD) (2018)

Soloists: Gerald Finley, Julia Bullock

Ensemble: BBC Symphony Orchestra, BBC Singers

Conductor: John Adams

DOCTOR ATOMIC SYMPHONY

Nonesuch 7559-79932-8 (CD) (2009)

Ensemble: Saint Louis Symphony Orchestra

Conductor: David Robertson

Chandos CHSA 5129 (CD) (2013)

Ensemble: Royal Scottish National Orchestra

Conductor: Peter Oundjian

EL DORADO

Nonesuch 7559-79359-2 (CD) (1996)

Ensemble: The Hallé Orchestra

Conductor: Kent Nagano

EL NIÑO

Nonesuch 7559-79634-2 (CD) (2001)

Ensembles: London Voices; Deutsches Symphonie-Orchester Berlin

Conductor: Kent Nagano

EROS PIANO

Nonesuch 7559-79249-2 (CD) (1991)

Soloist: Paul Crossley

Ensemble: Orchestra of St. Luke's

Conductor: John Adams

FEARFUL SYMMETRIES

Nonesuch 7559-79218-2 (CD) (1989)

Ensemble: Orchestra of St. Luke's

Conductor: John Adams

Actes Sud 34102 (CD) (1999)

Ensemble: Orchestre Philharmonique de Montpellier L.-R.

Conductor: René Bosc

CCn'C Records 01912 (CD) (2001)

Ensemble: Symphony Orchestra of Norrlands Opera

Conductor: Kristjan Järvi

FELLOW TRAVELER

Azica 71280 (CD) (2013)

Ensemble: Attacca Quartet

FIRST QUARTET

Azica 71280 (CD) (2013)

Ensemble: Attacca Quartet

Nonesuch 523014 (CD) (2011)

Ensemble: St. Lawrence String Quartet

GNARLY BUTTONS

Nonesuch 7559-79465-2 (CD) (1998)

Soloist: Michael Collins

Ensemble: London Sinfonietta

Conductor: John Adams

Virgin Classics 7243 5 45351 2 3 (CD) (1999)

Soloist: André Trouttet

Ensemble: Ensemble InterContemporain

Conductor: David Robertson

Divine Art 25138 (CD) (2017)

Soloist: Elizabeth Jordan

Ensemble: Northern Chamber Orchestra

Conductor: Stephen Barlow

GRAND PIANOLA MUSIC

EMI Angel Records CDC 7 47331 2 (CD) (1985)

Soloists: Alan Feinberg and Ursula Oppens, pianos

Ensemble: Solisti New York

Conductor: Ransom Wilson

Nonesuch 7559-79219-2 (CD) (1994)

Soloists: John Alley and Shelagh Sutherland, pianos

Ensemble: London Sinfonietta

Conductor: John Adams

Chandos 9363 (CD) (1995)

Soloists: Ellen Corver and Sepp Grotenhuis, pianos

Ensemble: Netherlands Wind Ensemble

Conductor: Stephen Mosko

SFS Media 0063 (CD) (2015)

Soloist: Orli Shaham and Marc-André Hamelin, pianos

Ensembles: San Francisco Symphony; Synergy Vocals

Conductor: John Adams

NEOS Music 21703 (CD) (2016)

Soloist: Andreas Grau and Götz Schumacher, pianos

Ensemble: Deutsches Symphonie-Orchester Berlin

Conductor: Brad Lubman

GUIDE TO STRANGE PLACES

Nonesuch 7559-79932-8 (CD) (2009)

Ensemble: Saint Louis Symphony Orchestra

Conductor: David Robertson

HALLELUJAH JUNCTION

Nonesuch 7559796992 (CD) (2004)

Soloist: Nicolas Hodges and Rolf Hind, piano

Black Box Classics 1098 (CD) (2005)

Soloists: James Ehnes and Andrew Russo, piano

Naxos American Classics 8.559285 (CD) (2007)

Soloists: Ralph van Raat and Maarten van Veen, piano

Turtle Records, TRSA 0021 (CD) (2008)

Soloists: Gerard Bouwhuis and Cees van Zeeland

Canary Classics 11 (CD) (2014)

Soloists: Orli Shaham and Jon Kimura Parker

Brilliant Classics 95388 (CD) (2017)

Soloists: Jeroen van Veen and Sandra van Veen

Skulpturenpark Waldfrieden CF 003 (CD) (2017)

Soloists: Holger Groschopp and Majella Stockhausen

HARMONIELEHRE

Nonesuch 7559-79115-2 (CD) (1985)

Ensemble: San Francisco Symphony

Conductor: Edo de Waart

Мелодия (Melodiya) A10 00477 004 (LP) (1989)

Ensemble: Lithuanian National Symphony Orchestra

Conductor: Juozas Domarkas

EMI Classics 7243 5 55051 2 (CD) (1994)

Ensemble: City of Birmingham Symphony Orchestra

Conductor: Simon Rattle

Arch Media 1014 (MP3) (2008)

Ensemble: Saint Louis Symphony Orchestra

Conductor: David Robertson

Prior Records 043/044 (CD) (2010)

Ensemble: Lithuanian National Symphony Orchestra

Conductor: Juozas Domarkas

SFS Media 0053 (CD) (2012)

Ensemble: San Francisco Symphony

Conductor: Michael Tilson Thomas

Chandos CHSA 5129 (CD) (2013)

Ensemble: Royal Scottish National Orchestra

Conductor: Peter Oundjian

HARMONIUM

ECM New Series 1277 (LP) (1984)

Ensembles: San Francisco Symphony Orchestra and Chorus

Conductor: Edo de Waart

Telarc Digital 80365 (CD) (1996)

Soloists: Renée Fleming, soprano; Karl Dent, tenor; Victor Ledbetter, baritone

Ensembles: Atlanta Symphony Orchestra and Chorus

Conductor: Robert Shaw

Nonesuch 79453-2 (10 CD Boxset) (1999)

Ensembles: San Francisco Symphony Orchestra and Chorus

Conductor: John Adams

Nonesuch 7559-79549-2 (CD) (2000)

Ensembles: San Francisco Symphony Orchestra and Chorus

Conductor: John Adams

BBC Music MM222 (CD) (2002)

Ensembles: BBC National Orchestra and Chorus of Wales

Conductor: Mark Elder

HOODOO ZEPHYR

Nonesuch 7559-79311-2 (CD) (1993)

Synthesizer: John Adams

I WAS LOOKING AT THE CEILING AND THEN I SAW THE SKY

Nonesuch 7559-79473-2 (CD) (1998)

Soloists: Audra McDonald, Michael McElroy, Welly Yang, Angela Teek, Darius de Haas, Marin Mazzie, Richard Muenz, vocals

Conductor: John Adams

Naxos 8.669003-04 (CD) (2005)

Ensembles: Young Opera Company Freiburg; The Band of Holst-Sinfonietta

Conductor: Klaus Simon

JOHN'S BOOK OF ALLEGED DANCES

Nonesuch 7559-79465-2 (CD) (1998)

Ensemble: Kronos Quartet

Analekta AN 2 8732 (CD) (2011)

Ensembe: La Pietà

Azica 71280 (CD) (2013)

Ensemble: Attacca Quartet

Skulpturenpark Waldfrieden CF 003 (CD) (2017)

Soloists: Liviu Neagu-Gruber, violin; Axel Hess, violin; Jens Brockmann, viola; Michael Hablitzel, cello

LA MUFA

Actes Sud OMA 34104 (CD) (1999)

Soloist: Jacques Prat

Ensemble: Orchestre Philharmonique de Montpellier L.-R.

Conductor: Enrique Diemecke

LE LIVRE DE BAUDELAIRE

BBC Music Magazine MM 239 (CD) (2004)

Soloist: Christopher Maltman, baritone

Ensemble: BBC Symphony Orchestra

Conductor: Thierry Fischer

Berlin Classics 0300832BC (CD) (2017)

Soloist: Christiane Karg, soprano

Ensemble: Bamberger Symphoniker

Conductor: David Afkham

LIGHT OVER WATER

New Albion 005 (LP) (1985)

Soloists: Brian McCarty, William Klingelhofer, French horn; John Adams, synthesizer; Don Kenelly, Mack Kenley, trombone; Jim Miller, Tim Wilson, trumpet; Zachariah Spellman, tuba

Conductor: John Adams

New Albion 014 (CD) (1987)

Soloists: Brian McCarty, William Klingelhofer, French horn; John Adams, synthesizer; Don Kenelly, Mack Kenley, trombone; Jim Miller, Tim Wilson, trumpet; Zachariah Spellman, tuba

LOLLAPALOOZA

BMG Classics/RCA Victor 09026-68798-2 (CD) (1998)

Ensemble: New World Symphony

Conductor: Michael Tilson Thomas

Nonesuch 79453-2 (10 CD Boxset) (1999)

Ensemble: The Hallé Orchestra

Conductor: Kent Nagano

Nonesuch 7559-79607-2 (CD) (2000)

Ensemble: The Hallé Orchestra

Conductor: Kent Nagano

MY FATHER KNEW CHARLES IVES

Nonesuch 7559-79857-2 (CD) (2006)

Ensemble: BBC Symphony Orchestra

Conductor: John Adams

NAIVE AND SENTIMENTAL MUSIC

Nonesuch 7559-79636-2 (CD) (2002)

Ensemble: Los Angeles Philharmonic

Conductor: Esa-Pekka Salonen

Chandos 5199 (CD) (2018)

Ensembles: Royal Scottish National Orchestra

Conductor: Peter Oundjian

NIXON IN CHINA

Elektra Nonesuch 7559-79177-2 (CD) (1988)

Ensembles: Orchestra and Chorus of St. Luke's

Conductor: Edo de Waart

Naxos 8.669022-24 (CD) (2009)

Soloists: Robert Orth, Maria Kanyova, Thomas Hammons, Marc Heller, Tracy Dahl, Chen-Ye Yuan

Ensemble: Colorado Symphony Orchestra and Opera Colorado Chorus

Conductor: Marin Alsop

ON THE TRANSMIGRATION OF SOULS

Nonesuch 7559-79816-2 (CD) (2004)

Ensembles: New York Philharmonic, Brooklyn Youth Chorus Academy, and New York Choral Artists

Conductor: Lorin Maazel

PHRYGIAN GATES

New Albion 007 (LP) (1986)

Soloist: Mack McCray

TROY 038 (CD) (1993)

Soloist: Christopher O'Riley

Music & Arts 862 (CD) (1995)

Solosit: Ursula Oppens

RCA Victor Red Seal 09026-68674-2 (CD) (1997)

Solosit: Hermann Kretzschmar

Tall Poppies 108 (CD) (1997)

Soloist: Peter Waters

Telarc 80513 (CD) (1998)
Soloist: Gloria Cheng-Cochran

Pianovox 510 (CD) (1998)
Soloist: Jay Gottlieb

Arabesque Recordings 6776 (CD) (2003)
Soloist: Bruce Brubaker

Nonesuch 7559796992 (CD) (2004)
Soloist: Rolf Hind, piano

Black Box Classics 1098 (CD) (2005)
Soloist: Andrew Russo

Stradivarius 33735 (CD) (2006)
Soloist: Emanuele Arciuli

Naxos American Classics 8.559285 (CD) (2007)
Soloist: Ralph van Raat, piano

ATMA Classique 22556 (CD) (2010)
Soloist: David Jalbert

Brilliant Classics 95388 (CD) (2017)
Soloist: Jeroen van Veen

ROAD MOVIES

Nonesuch 7559796992 (CD) (2004)
Soloist: Leila Josefowicz, violin; John Novacek, piano

Black Box Classics 1098 (CD) (2005)
Soloists: James Ehnes, violin; Andrew Russo, piano

Analekta AN 2 8732 (CD) (2011)
Ensembe: La Pietà
Soloists: Angèle Dubeau, violin; Louise Bessette, piano

Skulpturenpark Waldfrieden CF 003 (CD) (2017)

Soloists: Holger Groschopp, piano; Liviu Neagu-Gruber, violin

SAXOPHONE CONCERTO

Nonesuch 7559-79564-4 (CD) (2014)

Soloist: Timothy McAllister

Ensemble: St. Louis Symphony

Conductor: David Robertson

SCHEHERAZADE.2

Nonesuch 557170-2 (CD) (2016)

Soloist: Leila Josefowicz

Ensemble: St. Louis Symphony

Conductor: David Robertson

SCRATCHBAND

Etcetera KTC 9000 (CD) (2006)

Ensemble: Schönberg Ensemble

Conductor: John Adams

SHAKER LOOPS

1750 Arch Records S-1784 (LP) (1980)

Ensemble: The Ridge Quartet

Philips 412 214–1 (LP) (1984)

Ensemble: San Francisco Symphony

Conductor: Edo de Waart

New Albion 014 (CD) (1987)

Ensemble: The Ridge Quartet

Virgin Classics 7243 5 61121 2 4 (CD) (1994)

Ensemble: London Chamber Orchestra

Conductor: Christopher Warren-Green

BBC Radio Classics 15656 91692 (CD) (1996)

Ensemble: BBC Symphony Orchestra

Conductor: Richard Buckley

Nonesuch 7559-79360-2 (CD) (1996)

Ensemble: Orchestra of St. Luke's

Conductor: John Adams

RCA Victor Red Seal 09026-68674-2 (CD) (1997)

Ensemble: Ensemble Modern

Conductor: Sian Edwards

HMV Classics 7243 5 73040 2 (CD) (1998)

Ensemble: The London Chamber Orchestra

Conductor: Christopher Warren-Green

Naxos 8.559031 (CD) (2004)

Ensemble: Bournemouth Symphony Orchestra

Conductor: Marin Alsop

Oehms Classics OC 363 (CD) (2005)

Ensemble: Festival Strings Lucerne

Conductor: Achim Fiedler

Philips 475 7551 (CD) (2006)

Ensemble: San Francisco Symphony

Conductor: Edo de Waart

Analekta AN 2 8732 (CD) (2011)

Ensembe: La Pietà

Conductor: Angèle Dubeau

SHORT RIDE IN A FAST MACHINE: FANFARE FOR ORCHESTRA

Nonesuch 7559-79144-1 (LP) (1987)

Ensemble: San Francisco Symphony

Conductor: Edo de Waart

Nonesuch 7559-79144-2 (CD) (1987)

Ensemble: San Francisco Symphony

Conductor: Edo de Waart

EMI Classics 7243 5 55051 2 5 (CD) (1994)

Ensemble: City of Birmingham Symphony Orchestra

Conductor: Simon Rattle

Klavier Records KCD 11058 (CD) (1994)

Ensemble: Cincinnati Wind Symphony

Conductor: Eugene Corporon

Chandos CHAN 9636 (CD) (1995)

Ensemble: Netherlands Wind Ensemble

Conductor: Stephen Mosko

The Philharmonic-Symphony Society of New York NYP 9915 (CD) (1999)

Ensemble: New York Philharmonic

Conductor: Kurt Masur

BBC Music MM 222 (CD) (2002)

Ensemble: BBC National Orchestra of Wales

Conductor: Mark Elder

EMI Classics 7243 5 57129 2 9 (CD) (2002)

Ensemble: Philharmonisches Staatsorchester Hamburg

Conductor: Ingo Metzmacher

Naxos 8.559031 (CD) (2004)

Ensemble: Bournemouth Symphony Orchestra

Conductor: Marin Alsop

SFS Media 0053 (CD) (2012)
Ensemble: San Francisco Symphony
Conductor: Michael Tilson Thomas

Chandos CHSA 5129 (CD) (2013)
Ensemble: Royal Scottish National Orchestra
Conductor: Peter Oundjian

Mark Records 50916 (CD) (2015)
Ensemble: Florida Gulf Coast University Wind Orchestra
Conductor: Rod M. Chesnutt

Summit Records DCD 704 (CD) (2017)
Ensemble: Columbus State University Wind Ensemble
Conductor: Jamie L. Nix

SLONIMSKY'S EARBOX

Nonesuch 79453-2 (10 CD Boxset) (1999)
Ensemble: The Hallé Orchestra
Conductor: Kent Nagano

Nonesuch 7559-79607-2 (CD) (2000)
Ensemble: The Hallé Orchestra
Conductor: Kent Nagano

Q-Disc 97035 (CD) (2003)
Ensemble: North Netherlands Symphony Orchestra
Conductor: Jurjen Hempel

SON OF CHAMBER SYMPHONY

Nonesuch 7559-79800-8 (CD) (2011)
Ensemble: International Contemporary Ensemble
Conductor: John Adams

Cantaloupe Music CA21128 (CD) (2017)
Ensemble: Alarm Will Sound
Conductor: Alan Pierson

THE BLACK GONDOLA

Nonesuch 7559-79359-2 (CD) (1996)
Ensemble: London Sinfonietta
Conductor: John Adams

Jupiter Records 109 (CD) (2007)
Ensemble: London Symphony Orchestra
Conductor: Gisèle Ben-Dor

THE CHAIRMAN DANCES: FOXTROT FOR ORCHESTRA

Nonesuch 7559-79144-2 (CD) (1987)
Ensemble: San Francisco Symphony
Conductor: Edo de Waart

EMI Classics 7243 5 55051 2 (CD) (1994)
Ensemble: City of Birmingham Symphony Orchestra
Conductor: Simon Rattle

CCn'C Records 01912 (CD) (2001)
Ensemble: Symphony Orchestra of Norrlands Opera
Conductor: Kristjan Järvi

Decca CFM FW 119 (CD) (2009)
Ensemble: Hollywood Bowl Orchestra
Conductor: John Mauceri

THE DEATH OF KLINGHOFFER

Elektra Nonesuch 7559-79281-2 (CD) (1992)
Soloists: Sanford Sylvan, James Maddalena, and Sheila Nadler

Ensembles: The Orchestra of the Opéra de Lyon, The London Opera Chorus
Conductor: Kent Nagano

THE DEATH OF KLINGHOFFER CHORUSES

Nonesuch 7559-79549-2 (CD) (2000)
Ensembles: The Orchestra of the Opéra de Lyon, The London Opera Chorus
Conductor: Kent Nagano

THE DHARMA AT BIG SUR

Nonesuch 79857-2 (CD) (2006)
Soloist: Tracy Silverman
Ensemble: BBC Symphony Orchestra
Conductor: John Adams

Deutsche Grammophon 0289 477 9200 0 (MP3) (2010)
Soloist: Leila Josefowicz
Ensemble: Los Angeles Philharmonic
Conductor: John Adams

BBC Music MM406 (CD) (2016)
Soloist: Chloë Hanslip
Ensemble: BBC National Orchestra of Wales
Conductor: Eric Stern

THE GOSPEL ACCORDING TO THE OTHER MARY

Deutsche Grammophon 00289 479 2243 (CD) (2014)
Ensembles: Los Angeles Philharmonic and Master Chorale
Conductor: Gustavo Dudamel

THE WOUND-DRESSER

Nonesuch 7559-79218-2 (CD) (1989)
Soloist: Sanford Sylvan

Ensemble: Orchestra of St. Luke's

Conductor: John Adams

Late Junction BBCLJ30012 (CD) (2002)

Solosit: Christopher Maltman, baritone

Ensemble: BBC Symphony Orchestra

Conductor: John Adams

Naxos 8.559031 (CD) (2004)

Soloist: Nathan Gunn, baritone

Ensemble: Bournemouth Symphony Orchestra

Conductor: Marin Alsop

PentaTone Classics PTC 5186 393 (CD) (2011)

Soloists: Sanford Sylvan, baritone; Jun Iwasaki, violin

Ensemble: Oregon Symphony Orchestra

Conductor: Carlos Kalmar

Berliner Philharmoniker Recordings BPHR 170141 (CD) (2017)

Soloist: Georg Nigl, baritone

Ensemble: Berlinker Philharmoniker

Conductor: Kirill Petrenko

TODO BUENOS AIRES

TROY 509 (CD) (2002)

Soloist: Eric Segnitz, violin

Ensemble: Miramar Sinfonietta

Conductor: Henri B. Pensis

TROMBA LONTANA: FANFARE FOR ORCHESTRA

Nonesuch 7559-79144-2 (CD) (1987)

Ensemble: San Francisco Symphony

Conductor: Edo de Waart

EMI Classics 7243 5 55051 2 (CD) (1994)
Ensemble: City of Birmingham Symphony Orchestra
Conductor: Simon Rattle

Late Junction BBCLJ30012 (CD) (2002)
Soloists: Gareth Bimson, Martin Hurrell, trumpet
Ensemble: BBC Symphony Orchestra
Conductor: John Adams

VIOLIN CONCERTO

Nonesuch 7559-79360-2 (CD) (1996)
Soloist: Gidon Kremer
Ensemble: London Symphony Orchestra
Conductor: Kent Nagano

Telarc 80494 (CD) (1999)
Soloist: Robert McDuffie
Ensemble: Houston Symphony
Conductor: Christoph Eschenbach

Late Junction BBCLJ30012 (CD) (2002)
Soloist: Leila Josefowicz
Ensemble: BBC Symphony Orchestra
Conductor: John Adams

Naxos 8.559302 (CD) (2006)
Soloist: Chloë Hanslip
Ensemble: Royal Philharmonic Orchestra
Conductor: Leonard Slatkin

Naïve V 5368 (CD) (2014)
Soloist: Chad Hoopes
Ensemble: MDR Leipzig Radio Symphony Orchestra
Conductor: Kristjan Järvi

Signum Classics SIGCD468 (CD) (2016)

Soloist: Tamsin Waley-Cohen

Ensemble: BBC Symphony Orchestra

Conductor: Andrew Litton

Nonesuch 7559-79351-0 (CD) (2018)

Soloist: Leila Josefowicz

Ensemble: St. Louis Symphony Orchestra

Conductor: David Robertson

B

List of Compositions

STAGE WORKS (OPERA, MUSIC THEATER, ORATORIOS)

Title: *Nixon in China*

Media: opera (voice, orchestra)

Notes: composition won Grammy award in 1989

Year(s): 1985–1987

Libretto: Alice Goodman

Edition(s): Boosey & Hawkes, 1987

Premiere: October 22, 1987; Houston, Texas; Wortham Theater Center; Houston Grand Opera; John DeMain, conductor; Peter Sellars, director; Mark Morris, choreographer

Title: *The Death of Klinghoffer*

Media: opera (voice, orchestra)

Year(s): 1990

Libretto: Alice Goodman

Edition(s): Boosey & Hawkes

Premiere: March 19, 1991; Brussels; Théâtre de la Monnaie; Kent Nagano, conductor; Peter Sellars, director; Mark Morris, choreographer

Title: *I Was Looking at the Ceiling and Then I Saw the Sky*

Media: songplay (voice, orchestra)

Year(s): 1995

Libretto: June Jordan

Edition(s): Boosey & Hawkes

Premiere: May 3, 1995; University of California, Berkeley; Zellerbach Playhouse; Paul Drescher Ensemble; Grant Gershon, conductor; Peter Sellars, director

Title: *El Niño*

Media: oratorio (chorus, orchestra)

Year(s): 1999–2000

Text: Biblical texts, Gnostic Infancy Gospels, Sor Juana Inés de la Cruz, Rosario Castellanos

Edition(s): Boosey & Hawkes

Premiere: December 15, 2000; Châtelet, Paris; Deutsches Symphonie Orchester, London Voices; Kent Nagano, conductor; Peter Sellars, director; Dawn Upshaw, soprano; Lorraine Hunt-Lieberson, mezzo-soprano; Willard White, bass-baritone

Title: *Doctor Atomic*

Media: opera (voice, orchestra)

Year(s): 2004–2005

Libretto: Peter Sellars; drawn from original sources

Edition(s): Boosey & Hawkes

Premiere: October 1, 2005; San Francisco, California; San Francisco Opera House; Donald Runnicles, conductor; Peter Sellars, director; Gerald Finley, baritone; Kristine Jepson, mezzo-soprano

Title: *A Flowering Tree*

Media: opera (voice, orchestra)

Year(s): 2006

Libretto: John Adams and Peter Sellars; drawn from a South Indian folktale and poems translated by A.K. Ramanujan

Edition(s): Boosey & Hawkes

Premiere: November 14, 2006; Vienna, Austria; Orchestra Sinfónica Juvenil Simón Bolívar, Schola Cantorum de Venezuela; John Adams, conductor; Peter Sellars, director; Jessica Rivera, soprano; Russell Thomas, tenor; Eric Owens, baritone

Title: *The Gospel According to the Other Mary*

Media: oratorio (chorus, orchestra)

Year(s): 2012

Libretto: Peter Sellars, based on Old and New Testament sources

Edition(s): Boosey & Hawkes

Premiere: May 31, 2012; Los Angeles, California; Walt Disney Concert Hall; Los Angeles Philharmonic, Los Angeles Master Chorale; Gustavo Dudamel, conductor; Kelley O'Connor, mezzo-soprano; Tamara Mumford, contralto; Russell Thomas, tenor; Daniel Bubeck, counter-tenor; Brian Cummings, counter-tenor; Nathan Medley, counter-tenor

Title: *Girls of the Golden West*

Media: opera (voice, orchestra)

Year(s): 2017

Libretto: Peter Sellars, compiled from original sources

Edition(s): Boosey & Hawkes

Premiere: November 21, 2017; San Francisco, California; War Memorial Opera House; San Francisco Opera; Grant Gershon, conductor; Peter Sellars, director

ORCHESTRAL WORKS (SYMPHONIES, CONCERTI, VOICE AND ORCHESTRA)

Title: *Suite for String Orchestra*

Media: string orchestra

Notes: unpublished composition written with the aid of his composition teacher

Year(s): 1962

Premiere: 1962; New Hampshire State Hospital Auxiliary Orchestra

Title: *Overture in F*

Media: orchestra

Notes: unpublished composition; referenced in Adams's autobiography

Year(s): circa 1962

Title: *Common Tones in Simple Time*

Media: orchestra

Year(s): 1979

Edition(s): Associated Music Publishers, 1982

Premiere: January 30, 1980; San Francisco, California; Hellman Hall; San Francisco Conservatory of Music; John Adams, conductor

Title: *Shaker Loops*

Media: string orchestra version

Year(s):   1983

Edition(s): Associated Music Publishers

Premiere: April 1983; New York City; Alice Tully Hall; American Composers Orchestra; Michael Tilson Thomas, conductor

Title: *Harmonielehre*

Media: orchestra

Notes: nominated for the Pulitzer Prize

Year(s):   1984–1985

Edition(s): Associated Music Publishers, 1985

Premiere: March 21, 1985; San Francisco, California; Davies Hall; San Francisco Symphony; Edo de Waart, conductor

Title: *The Chairman Dances: Foxtrot for Orchestra*

Media: orchestra

Year(s):   1985

Edition(s): Associated Music Publishers, 1989

Premiere: January 31, 1986; Milwaukee, Wisconsin; Milwaukee Symphony; Lukas Foss, conductor

Title: *Tromba Lontana: Fanfare for Orchestra*

Media: orchestra

Year(s):   1986

Edition(s): Boosey & Hawkes

Premiere: April 4, 1986; Houston, Texas; Jones Hall; Houston Symphony; Sergiu Commissiona, conductor

Title: *Short Ride in a Fast Machine: Fanfare for Orchestra*

Media: orchestra

Year(s):   1986

Edition(s): Boosey & Hawkes

Premiere: June 13, 1986; Mansfield, Massachusetts; Pittsburgh Symphony Orchestra; Michael Tilson Thomas, conductor

Title: *The Nixon Tapes*

Media: voice and orchestra

Notes: scenes from *Nixon in China*

Year(s): 1987

Edition(s): Boosey & Hawkes

Premiere: July 7, 1998; Aspen, Colorado; Aspend Chamber Orchestra; John Adams, conductor

Title: *Fearful Symmetries*

Media: orchestra

Year(s): 1988

Edition(s): Boosey & Hawkes

Premiere: October 29, 1988; New York City; Avery Fisher Hall; Orchestra of St Luke's; John Adams, conductor

Title: *Eros Piano*

Media: piano and orchestra

Year(s): 1989

Edition(s): Boosey & Hawkes

Premiere: November 24, 1989; London, England; Queen Elizabeth Hall; London Sinfonietta; John Adams, conductor; Paul Crossley, piano

Title: *El Dorado*

Media: orchestra

Year(s): 1991

Edition(s): Boosey & Hawkes

Premiere: November 11, 1991; San Francisco, California; Davies Hall; San Francisco Symphony; John Adams, conductor

Title: *Violin Concerto*

Media: violin and orchestra

Year(s): 1993

Edition(s): Boosey & Hawkes

Premiere: January 19, 1994; Saint Paul, Minnesota; Ordway Music Theater; Minnesota Orchestra; Edo de Waart, conductor; Jorja Fleezanis, violin

Title: *Lollapalooza*

Media: orchestra

Year(s): 1995

Edition(s): Boosey & Hawkes

Premiere: November 10, 1995; Birmingham, England; City of Birmingham Symphony Orchestra; Simon Rattle, conductor

Title: *Gnarly Buttons*

Media: clarinet and small orchestra

Year(s): 1996

Edition(s): Boosey & Hawkes

Premiere: October 19, 1996; London, England; Queen Elizabeth Hall; London Sinfonietta; John Adams, conductor; Michael Collins, clarinet

Title: *Slonimsky's Earbox*

Media: orchestra

Year(s): 1996

Edition(s): Boosey & Hawkes

Premiere: September 12, 1996; Manchester, England; Bridgewater Hall; Halle Orchestra, Kent Nagano, conductor

Title: *Century Rolls*

Media: piano and orchestra

Year(s): 1997

Edition(s): Boosey & Hawkes

Premiere: September 25, 1997; Cleveland, Ohio; Severance Hall; Cleveland Orchestra; Christoph von Dohnányi, conductor; Emanuel Ax, piano

Title: *Naive and Sentimental Music*

Media: orchestra

Year(s): 1998–1999

Edition(s): Boosey & Hawkes

Premiere: February 19, 1999; Los Angeles, California; Dorothy Chandler Pavillion; Los Angeles Philharmonic Orchestra; Esa-Pekka Salonen, conductor

Title: *Guide to Strange Places*

Media: orchestra

Year(s):   2001

Edition(s): Boosey & Hawkes

Premiere: October 6, 2001; Amsterdam, Netherlands; The Royal Concertgebouw; Radio Filharmonisch Orkest; John Adams, conductor

Title: *My Father Knew Charles Ives*

Media: orchestra

Year(s):   2003

Edition(s): Boosey & Hawkes

Premiere: April 30, 2003; San Francisco, California; Davies Symphony Hall; San Francisco Symphony; Michael Tilson Thomas, conductor

Title: *The Dharma at Big Sur*

Media: electric violin and orchestra

Year(s):   2003

Edition(s): Boosey & Hawkes

Premiere: October 24, 2003; Los Angeles, California; Walt Disney Concert Hall; Los Angeles Philharmonic; Esa-Pekka Salonen, conductor; Tracy Silverman, violin

Title: *Doctor Atomic Symphony*

Media: orchestra

Year(s):   2007

Edition(s): Boosey & Hawkes

Premiere: August 21, 2007; London, England; Royal Albert Hall; BBC Symphony Orchestra; John Adams, conductor

Title: *City Noir*

Media: orchestra

Year(s):   2009

Edition(s): Boosey & Hawkes

Premiere: October 8, 2009; Los Angeles, California; Walt Disney Concert Hall; Los Angeles Philharmonic; Gustavo Dudamel, conductor

Title: *Absolute Jest*

Media: string quartet and orchestra

Year(s):   2011

Edition(s): Boosey & Hawkes

Premiere: March 15, 2012; San Francisco, California; Davies Symphony Hall; St Lawrence String Quartet; San Francisco Symphony; Michael Tilson Thomas, conductor

Title: *Saxophone Concerto*

Media: saxophone and orchestra

Year(s):   2013

Edition(s): Boosey & Hawkes

Premiere: August 22, 2013; Sydney, New South Wales; Sydney Opera House; Sydney Symphony Orchestra; John Adams, conductor; Timothy McAllister, saxophone

Title: *Scheherazade.2*

Media: violin and orchestra

Year(s):   2014

Edition(s): Boosey & Hawkes

Premiere: March 26, 2015; New York City; Avery Fisher Hall; New York Philharmonic; Alan Gilbert, conductor; Leila Josefowicz, violin

Title: *Must the Devil Have All the Good Tunes?*

Media: piano and orchestra

Year(s):   2019

Edition(s): Boosey & Hawkes

Premiere: March 7, 2019; Los Angeles; Walt Disney Concert Hall; Los Angeles Philharmonic; Gustavo Dudamel, conductor; Yuja Wang, piano

CHAMBER MUSIC

Title: *Piano Quintet*

Media: piano and strings

Notes: unpublished composition

Year(s): 1970

Premiere: May 1970; Cambridge, Massachusetts; John Knowles Paine Concert Hall, Harvard University; Luise Vosgerchian, piano; subsequently performed at the Marlboro Music Festival on August 20, 1970

Title: *Shaker Loops*

Media: string quartet

Notes: originally titled *Wavemaker*

Year(s): 1978

Edition(s): initially published by Associated Music Publisher but has been withdrawn from publication and replaced with the 1983 adaptation for string septet or string orchestra

Premiere: San Francisco, California; December 1978; Hellman Hall; New Music Ensemble of the San Francisco Conservatory; John Adams, conductor

Title: *Chamber Symphony*

Media: chamber orchestra

Year(s): 1992

Edition(s): Boosey & Hawkes

Premiere: January 17, 1993; The Hague; Netherlands; Dr. Anton Philipszaal; Schoenberg Ensemble; John Adams, conductor

Title: *John's Book of Alleged Dances*

Media: string quartet and pre-recorded CD

Year(s): 1994

Edition(s): Boosey & Hawkes

Premiere: November 19, 1994; Escondido, California; California Center for the Arts; Kronos Quartet

Title: *Road Movies*

Media: violin and piano

Year(s): 1995

Edition(s): Boosey & Hawkes

Premiere: October 23, 1995; Washington, D.C.; Kennedy Center; Robin Lorentz, violin; Vicki Ray, piano

Title: *Son of Chamber Symphony*

Media: chamber ensemble

Year(s):   2007

Edition(s):   Boosey & Hawkes

Premiere: November 30, 2007; Stanford, California; Dinkelspiel Auditorium; Alarm Will Sound; Alan Pierson, conductor

Title: *Fellow Traveler*

Media: string quartet

Year(s):   2007

Edition(s):   Boosey & Hawkes

Title: *First Quartet*

Media: string quartet

Notes: Adams's *First Quartet* represents the first multi-movement string quartet without a pre-recorded CD

Year(s):   2008

Edition(s):   Boosey & Hawkes

Premiere: January 29, 2009; New York City; Julliard School; Peter Jay Sharp Theater; St Lawrence String Quartet

Title: *Second Quartet*

Media: string quartet

Year(s):   2014

Edition(s):   Boosey & Hawkes

Premiere: January 18, 2015; Stanford, California; Stanford University; Bing Concert Hall; St Lawrence String Quartet

PIANO SOLO OR DUET

Title: *China Gates*

Media: piano

Notes: Adams's first piano piece is dedicated to pianist Sarah Cahill

Year(s):   1977

Edition(s):   Associated Music Publishers

Title: *Phrygian Gates*

Media: piano

Year(s): 1977–1978

Edition(s): Boosey & Hawkes

Premiere: March 17, 1978; San Francisco, California; Hellman Hall; Mack McCray, piano

Title: *Hallelujah Junction*

Media: piano

Year(s): 1998

Edition(s): Boosey & Hawkes

Premiere: April 3, 1998; Los Angeles, California; The Getty Center; Gloria Cheng and Grant Gershon, piano

Title: *American Berserk*

Media: piano

Year(s): 2001

Edition(s): Boosey & Hawkes

Premiere: February 25, 2002; New York City; Carnegie Hall; Garrick Ohlsson, piano

Title: *I Still Play*

Media: piano

Year(s): 2017

Edition(s): Boosey & Hawkes

Premiere: April 1, 2007; Brooklyn, New York; Peter Jay Sharp Building; Brooklyn Academy of Music; Jeremy Denk, piano

CHORAL WORKS

Title: *Ktaadn*

Media: piano and chorus

Notes: unpublished score; commissioned by Jon Bailey.

Year(s): 1972

Text: music set to the names of Abenaki towns including Millinocket, Pemadumcook, Mattawamkeag, Chesuncook, and others

Premiere: 1972; Berkeley, California; University of California Berkeley Art Museum

Title: *Harmonium*

Media: orchestra and chorus

Year(s):   1980–1981

Edition(s): Associated Music Publishers

Text: poetry by John Donne and Emily Dickinson

Premiere: April 16, 1981; San Francisco, California; Davies Hall; San Francisco Symphony Orchestra and Chorus; Edo de Waart, conductor

Title: *The Death of Klinghoffer Choruses*

Media: chorus and orchestra

Year(s):   1990

Edition(s): Boosey & Hawkes

Text: Alice Goodman

Title: *On the Transmigration of Souls*

Media: orchestra, chorus, children's chorus, and pre-recorded soundtrack

Notes: awarded the Pulitzer Prize in 2003

Year(s):   2002

Edition(s): Boosey & Hawkes

Text: derived from names of victims and missing persons

Premiere: September 19, 2002; New York City; Avery Fisher Hall; Brooklyn Youth Chorus and New York Choral Artists; New York Philharmonic; Lorin Maazel, conductor

TAPE AND ELECTRONIC COMPOSITIONS

Title: *Heavy Metal*

Media: tape composition using Adams's first synthesizer, the Studebaker

Notes: unpublished master's thesis; original master tape deteriorated beyond repair and no reproductions are in existence

Year(s):   1970

Title: *Schedules of Discharging Capacitors*

Media: homemade oscillators and band pass filters

Notes: unpublished composition

Year(s):   Adams asserts it was composed circa 1975

Title: *Studebaker*

Media: modular synthesizer featuring oscillators, filters and ring modulators

Notes: unpublished composition

Year(s):   circa 1976

Title: *Onyx*

Media: four-channel tape made on the Studebaker synthesizer

Notes: unpublished composition

Year(s):   circa 1976

Title: *Light Over Water*

Media: two-channel tape

Notes: Boosey & Hawkes; a revised version of *Available Light*;
recording available on New Albion 005

Year(s):   1983

Title: *Hoodoo Zephyr*

Media: MIDI keyboard

Year(s):   1992–1993

Edition(s):   composition not scored; recording available on Nonesuch 7559-79311-2

OTHER ENSEMBLE WORKS

Title: *Electric Wake*

Media: chamber ensemble

Notes: unpublished undergraduate thesis; the score is housed in the Eda Kuhn
Loeb Music Library at Harvard University

Year(s):   1969

Title: *American Standard*

Media: unspecified chamber ensemble and optional sound media

Notes: unpublished composition, except for the second movement, titled *Christian Zeal and Activity*

Year(s):   1973

Premiere: March 23, 1973; San Francisco, California; San Francisco Museum of Modern Art; San Francisco Conservatory New Music Ensemble; John Adams, conductor

Title: *Christian Zeal and Activity*

Media: chamber ensemble and pre-recorded tape

Notes: drawn from the second movement of *American Standard*

Year(s):   1973

Edition(s): Boosey & Hawkes

Premiere: March 23, 1973; San Francisco, California; San Francisco Museum of Modern Art; San Francisco Conservatory New Music Ensemble; John Adams, conductor

Title: *Grounding*

Media: voices, saxophones, and electronics

Year(s):   1975

Edition(s): Boosey & Hawkes

Premiere: November 1975; San Francisco, California; Hall of Flowers, Golden State Park; San Francisco Conservatory New Music Ensemble; John Adams, conductor

Title: *Lo-Fi*

Media: playing simultaneous 45- and 78-rpm records

Notes: aleatoric composition

Year(s):   unknown; thought to have been composed during the early 1970s.

Edition(s): Boosey & Hawkes Premiere: performed in the Hall of Flowers at Golden State Park

Title: *Grand Pianola Music*

Media: two pianos, three female voices, winds, brass, and percussion

Year(s):   1982

Edition(s): Associated Music Publishers

Premiere: February 6, 1982; San Francisco, California; Japan Center Theater; San Francisco Symphony; John Adams, conductor; Robin Sutherland and Julie Steinberg, piano

Title: *The Wound-Dresser*

Media: baritone and chamber orchestra

Year(s): 1988–1989

Text: poetry by Walt Whitman

Edition(s): Boosey & Hawkes

Premiere: February 24, 1989; Saint Paul, Minnesota; Saint Paul Chamber Orchestra; John Adams, conductor; Sanford Sylvan, baritone

Title: *Scratchband*

Media: amplified ensemble consisting of woodwinds, brass, two samplers, electric guitar, bass guitar, and percussion

Year(s): 1996

Edition(s): Boosey & Hawkes

Premiere: April 13, 1996; University Park, Pennsylvania; Pennsylvania State University; Ensemble Modern; John Adams, conductor

Title: *Nancy's Fancy*

Media: fanfare for brass and percussion

Notes: written as a tribute to Nancy H. Bechtle, former president of the San Francisco Symphony

Year(s): 2001

Edition(s): unpublished score

Premiere: December 2001; San Francisco, California; Davies Symphony Hall; San Francisco Symphony; Michael Tilson Thomas, conductor

ARRANGEMENTS, ORCHESTRATIONS, AND FILM SCORES

Title: *Matter of Heart*

Media: string ensemble and harp

Notes: original music composed for documentary film on the life of psychiatrist Carl G. Jung

Year(s):   1983

Edition(s): unpublished score; the documentary made by the video distributor Kino International

Title: *Berceuse élégiaque*

Media: chamber orchestra

Notes: Adams's arrangement of Busoni's *Berceuse élégiaque*

Year(s):   1989

Edition(s): Boosey & Hawkes

Premiere: June 8, 1989; Saint Paul, Minnesota; Saint Paul Chamber Orchestra; John Adams, conductor

Title: *The Black Gondola*

Media: orchestra or chamber orchestra

Notes: Adams's arrangement of Liszt's *La Lugubre Gondola II*

Year(s):   1989

Edition(s): Boosey & Hawkes

Premiere: October 27, 1989; Saint Paul, Minnesota; Ordway Center for Performing Arts; Saint Paul Chamber Orchestra; John Adams, conductor

Title: *Wiegenlied*

Media: orchestra or chamber orchestra

Notes: Adams's arrangement of Liszt's *Wiegenlied*

Year(s):   1989

Edition(s): Boosey & Hawkes

Title: *Le Livre de Baudelaire*

Media: voice and orchestra

Notes: Adams's arrangement of Debussy's *Cinq poèmes de Charles Baudelaire*

Year(s):   1993

Text: Charles Baudelaire

Edition(s): Boosey & Hawkes

Premiere: March 10, 1994; Amsterdam, Netherlands; Concertgebouw; The Royal Concertgebouw; Royal Concertgebouw Orchestra; John Adams, conductor; Robert Alexander, soloist

Title:	*La Mufa*
Media:	chamber orchestra
Notes:	Adams's arrangement of a tango by Astor Piazzolla.
Year(s):	1995
Edition(s):	Boosey & Hawkes
Premiere:	January 16, 1997; Cologne, Germany; Kölner Philharmonie; Deutsche Kammerphilharmonie Bremen; Gidon Kremer, violin

Title:	*Todo Buenos Aires*
Media:	violin and orchestra
Notes:	Adams's arrangement of a tango by Astor Piazzolla
Year(s):	1996
Edition(s):	Boosey & Hawkes
Premiere:	February 19, 1997; Heidelberg, Germany; Philharmonische Orchester Heidelberg; Thomas Kalb, conductor; Gidon Kremer, violin

Title:	*An American Tapestry*
Notes:	original music composed for documentary film on the American migration experience
Year(s):	1999
Edition(s):	unpublished score; documentary commissioned by and aired on the Showtime television channel

Title:	*Postmark (from Fearful Symmetries)*
Media:	soprano saxophone and piano
Notes:	arrangement by Marilyn Shrude
Year(s):	2009
Edition(s):	Boosey & Hawkes

Title:	*I Am Love*
Notes:	film score features pre-existing compositions by Adams; Luca Guadagnino, director; film producer and actress Tilda Swinton explains the film was created around Adams's compositions
Year(s):	2009
Film Distributor:	Magnolia Pictures

Title: *Shutter Island*

Notes: film score features Adams's *Christian Zeal and Activity*; Martin Scorsese, director; Leonardo DiCaprio, principal actor

Year(s):   2010

Film Distributor: Paramount Pictures

Title: *Roll Over Beethoven*

Media: two pianos

Notes: arrangement of Adams's 2014 *Second Quartet* by Preben Antonson

Year(s):   2014

Edition(s):   Boosey & Hawkes

Premiere: March 23, 2016; Greene Space, New York; Christina and Michelle Naughton, duo pianos

Title: *Call Me by Your Name*

Notes: film score features Adams's *Hallelujah Junction, China Gates*, and *Phrygian Gates*; Luca Guadagnino, director

Year(s):   2017

Film Distributor: Sony Pictures Classics

Title: *El Niño: A Paraphrase for Voices and Chamber Ensemble*

Notes: Selections from *El Niño* arranged by Preben Antonsen

Year(s):   2018

Edition(s):   Forthcoming through Boosey & Hawkes

C

Index of Authors

D

Index of Compositions and Arrangements

E

Subject Index

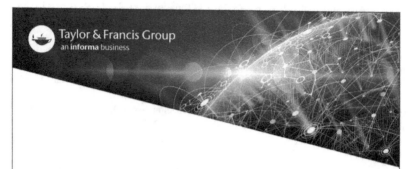